Living the Protein Lifestyle

Enjoy Better Health, Develop More Strength, and
Have More Energy!

Joshua D. Noland

JoshNoland.com

The stories and antidotes shared in this book are based on real people and situations. In some instances, names, places, and other details have been fictionalized to protect the anonymity of the people discussed.

The information given in this book should not be treated as a substitute for professional medical or clinical advice; always consult a medical or clinical practitioner. Any use of information in this book is at the reader's discretion and risk. Neither the author nor the publisher can be held responsible for any loss, claim, or damage arising out of the use or misuse of the suggestions made, the failure to take medical or clinical advice, or for any material on third-party websites.

WHY READ THIS BOOK

You will learn proven techniques I have developed and used personally to improve my physical and mental health. By following what is laid out in the chapters, you, too, can gain control of your health. I will tell you how I did it despite the challenges and reveal the key strategies you can use to find success and make lasting changes.

Your health is the determining factor to a long and happy life, so why not invest in yourself by gaining some knowledge that will help you feel and look your best? If you're confused about what you should be eating and doing for optimum health, this is the book for you.

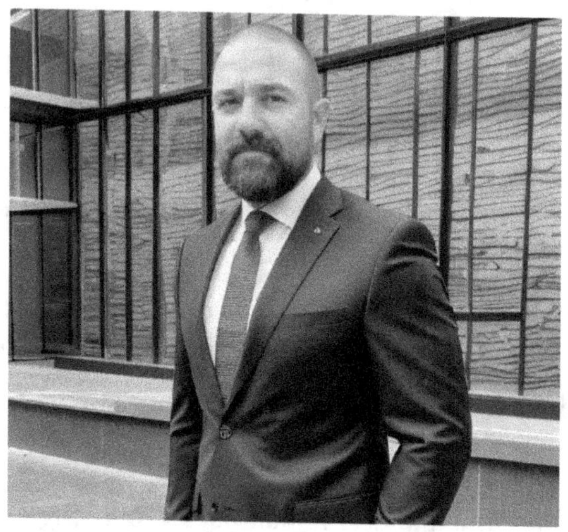

Joshua D. Noland is educated in the Science of Exercise at the University of Colorado Boulder and has studied food and health at Stanford University. His real-world experience in the food service industry has given him extensive inside knowledge of how foods are prepared and how to improve those methods. Sharing knowledge to help people overcome their health struggles is his passion. Josh also enjoys the outdoors and is an avid dog lover. Visit his website at JoshNoland.com to learn more about him and to get his top three high-protein, easy-to-make recipes to kick-start your health journey today!

TABLE OF CONTENTS

CHAPTER 1:
HOW PROTEIN CHANGED MY LIFE

Eating more protein was the ultimate key to my long-term health success. Over the span of two years I slowly started taking control of my health, but when I started incorporating more protein into my diet everything got a whole lot easier. I felt good, looked better, and had more energy to do the things I had to do and I started living my best life.

a. Overweight, depressed, feeling stuck, and lots of bad habits. That was me in 2019. I was eating, drinking, and smoking too much and I felt like shit. I was so out of shape; it was hard to tie my shoes, I would be out of breath as if I had just run a marathon after only walking up a few steps. I was struggling physically and mentally; I was miserable and needed help. I didn't know where to start, nor did I have the strength to make a change on my own.

b. One day, out of the blue, my wife said that she'd signed up for a fitness challenge.

    "That's awesome!" I said.

    "Thanks. It's a six-week health challenge for women, and the winner gets $200."

    "I'm really proud and excited for you!" I desperately wanted to join her to show my support, but I was not ready. I did not have a lack of motivation—I had none. After watching her lose twenty pounds and feeling proud of what she was doing, I was inspired to give it a try. *Why not?* I thought. *What do I have to lose?*

I wasn't ready to change the way I was eating quite yet, but I was ready to make a change because I was not happy with how I looked and felt. I started working out a couple of days a week with my wife, but that didn't last long. We were at different levels of fitness, and I am very vocal. When I was pushing myself through a tough exercise, I would grunt and breathe loudly, so we agreed to continue exercising but not at the same time.

At first, working out was really difficult for me because I would get winded so fast that I felt like a loser. I didn't have a lot of stamina, but I kept trying, and after a few weeks, I noticed I could do more repetitions without having to take so many breaks because I was breathing better and getting stronger.

I also started talking to a therapist around that time, and one of the things they recommended was trying meditation. I had never thought of myself as that type of person, but I was open to trying new things to change my state of mind, so I tried it. I started meditating every morning and discovered that I liked it. I felt empowered because it gave me a chance to clear my head and set a positive tone for the day.

After about a month of working out and meditating, I was starting to feel pleased with my progress, and I felt the urge to start changing my eating habits. Now, I did not go cold turkey, give up all the junk food, and become a full-blown carnivore because that would have been too much of a drastic change, but I did start to change the way I ate. I still desperately craved junk food like Flamin' Hot Cheetos and chocolate ice cream (chocolate is my kryptonite). The cravings for junk food were so strong that I would feel comfort just knowing I had a bag of Cheetos at home to munch on later while sitting on the couch watching a movie.

I allowed myself to continue to eat junk food, but I started eating less and replacing it with healthier options like homemade popcorn. When you make popcorn at home, you are in control of how much oil and salt you use, so I used less of both to make it a better snack option.

I started eating more whole foods like meat, vegetables, fruits, and nuts. After a few weeks, my cravings shifted. I noticed that I wanted more meat and whole foods in general and less processed junk food.

By now, I was really getting into my health, so I started educating myself on the subject. I took an online course on the science of exercise and nutrition, and I started listening to science-based health and fitness-related podcasts. I discovered that protein is the most important macronutrient for overall health because it is used to build and repair every cell in your body, and most people are not eating enough. (I will occasionally refer to macronutrients as macros throughout the book.)

If you eat the proper amount of protein to hit your specific goals and body type, you will be less likely to overeat because it is so satiating.

I started including more protein in my meals, specifically animal protein. I noticed that I felt fuller for longer and had more energy throughout the day. I started to notice that when I overconsumed carbohydrates (carbs), especially those rich in gluten like pasta or bread, I felt sluggish and sleepy afterward. On the other hand, when I opted for a protein-heavy meal, I felt satiated and devoid of any adverse side effects.

The experts in the fitness industry say you should eat one gram of protein per pound of your ideal body weight to maintain and grow muscle. However, there are a lot of factors that go into determining the proper ratio of macronutrients for your body. Most people under-consume protein and have no idea what it can do to improve their health, especially if they're trying to lose weight, build muscle, or simply improve their overall health.

My ideal body weight is 180 pounds, meaning I need to eat 180 grams of protein per day as a general rule to nourish my body properly. If you have ever tracked your food intake, you know that it is a lot of protein! Don't fret. I will share with you some of the creative ways I have used to bump up my protein intake in later chapters of this book.

How much protein are you consuming every day? Are you eating enough? Do you eat mostly whole or processed foods? What does your diet look like? When I say "diet," I don't mean a time-bound scheme someone is advertising for fast weight loss. Your diet is simply the type of foods and drinks you regularly consume. Do you primarily eat plant or animal-based proteins? The difference can have a significant impact on how you look and feel.

In this book, I will share with you how, when you eat the proper amount of protein, you will naturally start to make healthier food choices, feel better, and have more energy. I will discuss such topics as animal versus plant-based protein, how eating more protein improved my life and the small but critical methods I use every day to achieve health success. I will help you learn how to consume the appropriate amount and the right kind of protein, whether you're at home or on the go. I refer to this as Living the Protein Lifestyle; it's not a diet, it's a lifestyle. Do you know why it's critical to eat your protein first at each meal? Keep reading, and you'll soon find out.

Everyone is different. For me, I had to start exercising before I could start making better food choices because I am an emotional eater. When I felt stressed out, depressed, or tired, I would eat foods I liked to help deal with those feelings. I would also eat those foods to celebrate. I would go all out and eat until I was stuffed. Once I felt better about my body, I was able to change my eating habits, and I started to reduce the amount and frequency of my drinking and smoking habits.

You may have more success by changing what you eat first, and then you may be more motivated and/or have the energy to exercise. You need to try different things and find what works for you. One important thing to remember when trying to improve your health is to make small changes. If you try to make too many changes at once, it can be overwhelming, and you will be more likely to give up. Everyone is different, so keep trying new things to see what works for you.

Before I started my health journey, I ate all kinds of junk food like chips and candy, but not too long after I started incorporating more protein into my diet and exercising, I began craving that stuff less and less, and I started snacking on healthier choices like dates with peanut butter covered in dark chocolate or fresh blueberries in the evenings. No one is perfect, but as long as you attempt to make healthier choices, you will be better off. If you mess up one day, it's okay; you can try again the next. You can exercise all you want, but you will never be able to burn more calories than you can consume.

I started adding more protein to my diet slowly by eating an extra egg or three in the morning and adding whey protein shakes to my daily regimen. I subscribed to Butcher Box so that high-quality meat would magically show up at my door; it was one less thing to have to worry about. I also started to focus my meals around protein and fill in the rest with vegetables and leafy greens. It was quite an adjustment to be eating so much meat, but these protein-centric meals would keep me full between meals but not make me feel lethargic.

I try to get all the protein my body requires by being aware of my daily protein goals, having high-protein foods and snacks on hand, and doing a bit of planning. I plan my meals ahead of time as much as possible and have figured out several tips for eating high protein on the go; both will be discussed in their own chapters in the book. I have also developed a ton of recipes, some of which I will share with you.

Once I implemented a high-protein diet, it helped limit my intake of highly processed foods and stop overeating because my body was getting all the nutrients it needed, and I felt satiated. Eventually, those processed food cravings disappear, and your body will start craving whole foods. I lost fifty pounds in the two years after starting my health journey, and I have maintained a healthy weight ever since by focusing on eating protein first and doing something physically active every day.

By continuing to read this book and implementing just some of the suggestions offered, I promise you will notice a difference. You will feel better, have more energy, and suffer less from noncontagious diseases like diabetes and obesity. Protein is not a miracle solution to all your problems, but if you are under-consuming it, your health will suffer. Your nutrition plays a significant part in how you look and feel, and when you combine that with a daily dose of exercise, you will be amazed at the results. If you stick with it and don't cheat yourself, you will be amazed at your results. You can do this!

I'll educate you on the science-based research and why you should be eating animal-based protein. I will help guide you on how to increase your protein intake. I'll discuss why it is also important to exercise and move your body every day. Life is chaotic, and it's a challenge to get all the nutrients you need, but with just a few of the tips you will learn in this book, you will get a handle on it and can even thrive as a human being in the frenzied world we inhabit today. I am confident that if you follow what I discuss in this book, you will find long-lasting success.

CHAPTER 2:
KNOWING IS HALF THE BATTLE: THE REMAINDER REQUIRES DEDICATION AND EFFORT

It was a sweltering, sunny summer day in the San Fernando Valley. The sweat was dripping down my face. I had replaced the ice in the beverage tub three times already. "Let's start packing up. It's too hot out here," I told Tony. We finally started loading up the truck. I went to pick up an ice chest off the ground, and when I lifted it up, it felt like a lightning bolt shot through my lower back. I wanted to go home already and take a cold shower, but I kept working. The next morning, the pain was so excruciating I could not get out of bed.

I tried resting for a few weeks, but my back did not seem to be getting any better, and that lightning started shooting down my right leg, so against all my manly intuition, I went to see my doctor. I got an x-ray, but it didn't show anything, so I got a magnetic resonance imaging scan (MRI). The doctor called me and said, "You have a bulging disc in your lower back, and you have two options. You can get surgery or try physical therapy." He went on to say, "I do not recommend this type of intensive surgery for someone your age; it should only be a last resort because there is no guarantee you will be pain-free. The pain could be worse, and you would have reduced mobility in your back for the rest of your life."

"Well, it sounds like I should try physical therapy."

"I will put in the authorization, and here is a prescription for oxycodone for the pain."

After a few months of physical therapy, my back was still sensitive. I could not sit for long or do anything that impacted my spine without the shooting pains returning. The pain medication was not helping with the pain anymore, so the doctor decided to put me on a pain management medication called methadone, a hard-core drug used to manage pain and help heroin addicts kick their addictions. If you've ever had any experience with these kinds of drugs, you know they are serious. They took the edge off, but I could not do much while on them, and then there was the constipation. After about a month of this, I decided it was too much. I wanted to take back control of my life, so I weaned myself off the drugs and started swimming and working out every day at the local YMCA.

After a few weeks, my back started feeling a bit better, so I slowly started hiking and getting into other low-impact outdoor activities. My back got stronger day by day; I even dropped a few pounds, and I was feeling good about myself.

This went on for a few years. Then I met my wife-to-be, got busy working an office job, and stopped being as active. This led to me putting on the weight I had lost plus some.

I believe I was not able to stay at a healthy weight long-term because I did not incorporate the changes I could have made into my lifestyle. The key I missed back then was to change my eating habits and stick with being physically active every day.

Doctors are trained to diagnose symptoms, and they only have two ways to treat them: by prescribing medications or surgery. They do not look at the problem from a holistic viewpoint to find the root problem. The way our healthcare system works here in the US, doctors do not have the time necessary to get to know their patients and get the whole picture. When you eat the right food for your body—in appropriate amounts—it will go a long way in healing a lot of common health issues and noncontagious diseases. "Let food be thy medicine." I think there is truth to that saying. I think, food can be a preventative medicine if you eat the right kind.

Everyone has been on a diet or three at one time or another. There are so many out there that it's overwhelming to know which ones are right for you. Most of these diets are not sustainable, but some of them are on the right track. Some mainstream diets work for certain applications. A one-day juice cleanse may be a good way to get a fresh start on a new diet and detoxify your body, or a thirty-day carnivore diet could be used as an elimination diet to help you figure out what foods your body does not respond well to. It could also help reduce cravings for unhealthy foods. Cravings have been attributed to your gut bacteria, and if you stop eating a food, the bacteria that fed on that food will starve, and your cravings will be reduced. Your daily intake should include foods you enjoy and exclude foods your body doesn't respond well to.

Common diets that work but are not be sustainable:

- Mediterranean diet: Whole foods, like fruits, vegetables, whole grains, lean proteins, and healthy fats, are influenced by the types of food eaten in cultures near the Mediterranean Sea.

- Keto diet: A low-carb, high-fat diet that gets you into a state of ketosis where the body burns fat for energy.

- Paleo diet: Only eat foods that people ate in the Paleolithic era, like lean meats, fish, fruits, vegetables, nuts, and seeds, while avoiding processed foods, dairy, and grains.

- Whole30: A 30-day elimination diet that restricts processed foods, added sugars, grains, dairy, and legumes to reset eating habits and identify food sensitivities.

- Intermittent fasting: Not really a diet but a schedule of when to and when not to eat.

These diets all have good aspects to them but can be challenging or detrimental to long-term success. For example, fasting can be a great way to reset your gut and reduce inflammation that can lead to autoimmune diseases; nonetheless, if you do it every day, you may struggle to eat enough calories. Keto can be helpful to burn fat, but you can't stay in ketosis forever, and this type of diet may be too fat-focused for your body type. Your diet should consist mostly of animals and plants that have been minimally processed, as well as foods you enjoy eating. The key is to mostly eat whole foods, avoid foods that you are sensitive to, and allow yourself to eat the other stuff once in a while, and do not be too hard on yourself if you get off track from time to time.

When early humans came out of the trees and started hunting and eating more meat, it caused our brains to grow, and I believe that has played a huge role in transforming us from our common ancestors into modern-day humans. Most people are not eating enough of or the right types of protein, which has had detrimental repercussions on our society's health.

Proteins I recommend:

- Beef

- Chicken

- Fish

- Eggs

As far as proteins go, not all are created equally. There are animal and plant-based proteins, and I believe animal protein is the superior source because it is nutrient-dense, bioavailable, and contains all nine essential amino acids. Even processed meats are not the same as whole cuts of meat; they taste good but are not the best for you because they may contain unhealthy preservatives and lots of sodium. Try to limit the amount of processed meats you eat to maximize your health.

Examples of processed meats:

- Pepperoni

- Hot dogs

- Deli meats

- Beef jerky

It drives me crazy to see how poorly some animals are treated, so much so that in 2014, I took a forty-hour permaculture design course in Ojai, California, to learn how to raise animals and grow plants in a more natural and sustainable way. If you have never heard of permaculture, it is a design science focused on living in a way that has a positive impact on the environment with the least amount of input over time. If you want to learn more, search for Geoff Lawton online and watch some of his YouTube videos.

As far as raising animals with love and care, there are humane ranchers out there who treat their livestock with respect. I feel if they can provide a good quality of life for an animal, then that animal will only have one bad day, and we get the benefit of consuming the most nutrient-dense food on the planet. Sustainable and humane animal operations offer better options to get high-quality meat without negatively impacting our environment or the life of the animal.

Most people don't know how important protein is to a healthy functioning body and how it can help you get a hold of your eating habits. I believe if I had started eating more protein when recovering from my back injury, I could have healed faster and kept the weight off for good. Even if you know the right foods to eat, it's hard to put that knowledge into practice because we're all busy with life, but if you want to live a long and happy life, you must stop and take control. That's why I'm so excited to share the tips and tricks I use to seamlessly incorporate more protein into your diet.

Protein can help you lose fat and gain lean body mass. It's not just for bodybuilders or weight lifters; it's for everyone. Even your grandparents can benefit from an increased protein intake. No matter what types of foods you like, you can always find a way to add more protein to each meal by making an informed choice. An increase in protein consumption, in addition to resistance training, will help you gain strength, stronger bones, and stability. This is critical for everyone, but especially for our aging population, to avoid injuries. If you want to stay mobile in your later years, start now. It's never too late.

If you want to lose weight, eating more protein is the best way to lose body fat and mitigate the amount of lean body mass (muscle) you lose. If you can incorporate additional protein into your regular diet, you will not be as hungry because protein takes longer to digest, so you feel fuller for longer and, as a side effect, you'll have less room in your stomach to overeat carbs. Carbs then can be converted to sugar and ultimately stored as fat if you don't use up all that potential energy with physical activity, and it takes a lot to burn off all those calories you get from overeating carbs. With most people working a desk job and or living a sedentary lifestyle due to too much screen time, this is often the case and why so many people are overweight these days.

I am not selling a diet. I am offering you the idea that *your lifestyle and habits will ultimately determine your health*. I am only offering the truth because there is so much bullshit out there that it's hard to know who to trust, and I hope to earn your trust and help you. Following a diet to strictly lose weight is not sustainable. You will get burned out and quit if you're too strict with yourself. You must develop healthy food habits and incorporate daily exercise into your lifestyle to make a long-lasting change.

Many people are confused about what foods are good for their bodies, and the reason is misinformation for the sole purpose of corporate profits. Food companies have been conducting studies for a long time, and when the data shows that their products are not good for your health, they tend to manipulate the data to make their products look better.

For example, according to an article in *JAMA Internal Medicine* posted in November 2016 called "Sugar Industry and Coronary Heart Disease Research: A Historical Analysis of Internal Industry Documents,"[1] the Sugar Research Foundation funded a study that showed that sugar was not bad for you and that fat was to blame for coronary heart disease. This is a flat-out lie and has played a huge role in misinformation; this is why people were unaware of how bad sugar is for you and why they are still afraid to eat dietary fat.

Another example is the American food guide pyramid. The food lobbyists had a lot of power, as most lobbyists still

---

[1] C. E. Kearns, L. A. Schmidt, & S. A. Glantz. "Sugar Industry and Coronary Heart Disease Research: A Historical Analysis of Internal Industry Documents." *JAMA Intern Med.* 2016; 176(11):1680–1685.

do today, and the US government was pressured to make grains the base of the pyramid, which suggested to people that's where the majority of their calories should come from.

This is straight-out misinformation, and if you follow it, you will have a tough time staying healthy. For years, the government and doctors told you fat was bad and grains were good but that is not the whole truth. There are different types of fat—some good, some bad—and the same goes for grains. What is certain is that six to eleven servings a day of bread, cereals, rice, and pasta, as recommended in the food pyramid, are simply way too much and won't leave room for enough of that essential protein.

Have you ever gone out to eat and found it hard to make healthy food choices? Do you know what foods your body responds negatively to? It's so hard to eat a balanced meal these days when you're out at a restaurant because the meals are usually not well-balanced in terms of proteins, starches, and vegetables, especially fast food. French fries are probably one of the worst foods, and they are super-addicting. McDonald's fries used to be fried in beef tallow, which is a much better fat than the canola oil they use now, but you should always limit the amount of fried foods you eat no matter what kind of oil is used. Even if you know what foods to avoid, you have to take the time to think and plan out your meals in advance to stay on track.

With the internet and social media, there is so much information available, and it can be confusing to know what foods you should or should not be eating. I struggled for years with this, and to be honest, I still do. It's overwhelming. There are just too many people with opposing ideas. That's why I stick with science-based information and research when it comes to nutrition.

According to data from the Centers for Disease Control,[2] the prevalence of obesity among adults in the United States was 42.4 percent in 2018, the most recent year for which data is available. This means that almost half of all the adults in the United States have a body mass index (BMI) of thirty or higher. I'm sure this number is way higher now after we were all locked down in our homes during the COVID crisis—uncertain of the future, deprived of socialization, and depressed. Those circumstances will make almost anyone eat more and be less motivated to take care of themselves. I, however, was lucky enough to have a set of weights at home and was able to use that time to focus on my health. I knew the healthier I was, the better chance my body had to fight any disease that came my way.

Si se puede is a Spanish saying that I love; it means "Yes, you can," and I know you can do this. You have the power to take control of your life, specifically your physical and mental health. Your health is the most important thing if you want to live a long and joyful life. You are already headed in the right direction by reading this book. All you have to do now is continue reading and put what you learn into action. I do not have formal training, but I have found success personally by experimenting with different strategies. I'm going to share the beneficial ones with you because I want to help you be your best self. It's not easy, but it's achievable. *Si se puede.*

---

[2] C. M. Hales, M.D. Carroll, C. D. Fryar, & C.L. "Prevalence of Obesity and Severe Obesity among Adults: United States, 2017–2018. NCHS Data Brief, no 360. Hyattsville, MD: National Center for Health Statistics. 2020

You may be asking yourself, *How can I eat healthy if I'm always so busy, always being pulled in so many directions by life?* This is a common struggle in our fast-paced society. Between work, socializing, and taking care of your other responsibilities, it can be hard to find the time. Unfortunately, it takes time and energy to make the right food choices to optimize your health, but I will discuss in future chapters how meal prepping can save the day when you don't have time during the week. I'll share tips for eating clean on the go and how to customize meal options at restaurants to make them more optimal. Some of the common questions you may be asking are addressed here:

Am I too old to start now? Has the opportunity passed me by? The answer is a resounding no. It's never too late to start eating right and gaining control of your health. You will have to do more than just eat right. The older we get, the more important it is to stay active. If you live a sedentary lifestyle, you'll need to start slow and build your strength, but once you get there, you'll need to stay active and continue eating properly to avoid noninfectious diseases and keep your body's immune system in a state to better defend against those infectious ones. I recently learned that what we know as Alzheimer's and dementia are really type 3 diabetes mellitus (T3DM) caused by consuming too much sugar. This is also known as diabetes of the brain.

What if I'm a picky eater? How can I be successful? If you fall into this category, you'll have to put in a little more effort to find foods you like that also have a higher protein content. No matter what types of foods you like, there are always options. For example, protein shakes could be plant- or whey-based, and when you start exploring all the different flavor combinations, the sky's the limit. The internet is filled with protein shake recipes if you have trouble thinking of some on your own. You must dedicate a bit of time every day and be open to trying new things to make this work.

What if I don't know how to cook? It's never too late to start learning to cook or prepare simple meals at home. There are so many videos on how to cook online and recipes to give you ideas. If you just take the time to learn and start slowly, you can succeed. I will share some of my recipes with you in later chapters of this book. Cooking at home is more cost-effective than eating out or buying prepared meals. If you absolutely cannot cook due to a lack of knowledge or your living situation, there are alternative solutions for you, and I will also discuss those solutions in further chapters.

I love animals and would never consider eating them; how do I get enough protein? Not all ranching practices are the same; some ranchers care about the quality of life of their animals and want them to be happy. They graze them on natural foods like grass and treat them with respect. Those lucky animals only have one bad day. If there is absolutely no way in hell you would ever eat the flesh of another animal, you can get the nutrition your body needs from plants, but it will be harder and take more planning and preparation, but it is possible.

Protein is an essential macronutrient required for the proper functioning of the human body. It's crucial for building and repairing tissues, maintaining healthy bones, producing hormones and enzymes, and transporting oxygen throughout the body. A case study on the impact of eating protein on health was conducted with a thirty-five-year-old female who had a sedentary lifestyle and was not consuming enough protein.

Before starting the study, the patient underwent a complete physical examination, which revealed low muscle mass, weakness, and fatigue. The patient's daily protein intake was recorded, and it was found that she was consuming only 40 grams of protein per day, which was well below the recommended daily minimum intake of 0.36 grams of protein per pound of body weight.

The patient was advised to increase her protein intake by consuming protein-rich foods such as meats, fish, eggs, beans, and nuts. After three months of following the recommended diet, the patient's muscle mass had significantly improved, and her fatigue had reduced. She also reported feeling more energetic and could easily perform daily activities.

In addition, the patient's blood test results showed an increase in hemoglobin levels, indicating an improvement in oxygen transport throughout the body. The patient's bone density also improved, reducing the risk of osteoporosis.

However, it is essential to note that excessive protein intake can lead to health problems in susceptible individuals, like people with poor kidney function. Therefore, it is important to consume the recommended amount of protein, maintain a balanced diet, and exercise daily.

In conclusion, the case study highlights the significant positive impact of eating protein on overall health, including muscle mass, bone density, and energy levels. It also emphasizes the importance of consuming the recommended daily protein intake and maintaining a balanced diet to avoid any adverse health effects.

The case study above proves my point. If all you did was start consuming more protein today without exercising or watching your carb intake, you will naturally start to feel better, and your health will improve. Now, if you start working out and/or going for daily walks and consuming more protein, you will notice the health benefits much faster. I promise you, if you take this information seriously and begin to implement some of the strategies I'm sharing, you will get stronger, feel better, and get more joy out of your life. Building more muscle mass alone will help with many things, like burning more calories in your daily activities and help you avoid injuries.

Knowing is half the battle, and I will help teach you what you need to know to start taking care of your body, but the remainder requires dedication and effort that will need to come from you. Now you have an idea of what an increase in protein can do for you, so get on it and add some extra protein to your next meal so you can start to experience the protein lifestyle for yourself.

CHAPTER 3:
FINDING BALANCE AND EMBRACING MODERATION

I never saw myself as a fit person growing up. I've always loved food and ate for pleasure. "You should eat to fuel your body, not for pleasure" is the saying I often heard. But food is just so good. That concept never clicked with me until a few years ago; even now, I look forward to eating my favorite foods and trying new ones.

The difference now is that I go out of my way to find foods I like that are good for me, and simultaneously, I limit the amount of foods I eat that I know are not the best for my health, like processed foods. Eating the foods you love, especially with loved ones, is one of the best parts of life, but moderation is the key to being happy and fit.

I have seen the positive effects an increase in protein consumption has had on me, and I know that eating enough protein and whole foods in general can have a positive impact on you, too. Of course, there will be challenges, but if you want to be successful, you need to start slow and stick with it to see results. There will be setbacks, but as long as you realize you're off track and get back on, you will do fine.

I am so excited to share with you how I formed long-lasting healthy habits in my life and offer these solutions to help you do the same. Protein is not a miracle food, and there is hard work involved, but knowing the information I am about to unfold in the following chapters is the key to your success as long as you can stick with it and make small changes over time. I do not have all the answers, but I have a few, and I have found personal success by utilizing them.

Decoding Nutrition

We all took it in high school, or most of us did, but that was a while ago for me, so a refresher is in order. In this chapter, I will touch on why it is essential to eat whole proteins, where to find them, how to make them by combining different foods, and some examples.

I know it is challenging to avoid processed foods since they are so abundant and convenient. However, I will discuss the reasons why you should limit how much you eat and why, when you eat mostly whole foods, you are setting yourself up for success. I will also review how different foods affect your blood sugar levels, how to identify foods that will spike your blood sugar levels easily, and how cholesterol got a bad rap but is actually critical for healthy brain function and many other functions in the body.

Not All Proteins Are Created Equally

Sometimes, two things can appear the same on the outside but are very different inside; for example, factory-farmed versus pasture-raised chicken. The factory-farmed chicken lives a horrible existence of overcrowding and living in an unnatural environment. The stress, antibiotics, and commercial feeds all have negative effects on the end product. On the flip side, pasture-raised chickens eat a more natural diet, breathe fresh air, and are exposed to sunlight. These two differently raised chickens may look similar at a glance, but the pasture-raised chicken will always be superior in the nutrient density of its meat and is overall healthier due to a low stress and natural environment.

The same goes for plant-based proteins like soy and peas. Organically grown plants are better than commercial farming operations because they use fewer chemicals to kill weeds and pests. The best option by far is homegrown, for sure. It's the only way to really know what was used in the growing and harvesting processes.

You Cannot Change What You Do Not Measure

Knowing what to eat and how much will drastically improve the odds of your success, but if you do not have a way to measure and keep track of the foods and quantities you eat, you won't be able to adjust or stay within your goals. It's not just about protein or calories. When you start to eat to fuel your body, you will need to track everything you eat and be accurate in your measurements, like a scientist, if you want accurate results. This takes a little effort and a scale, but keeping a food journal will help you know where you are and what direction you need to go regarding your eating habits. I will discuss tips I use daily to help me stay on track and how you can, too. I will also share which apps I use and how you can create shortcuts to streamline your food tracking.

Home Cooking: A Recipe for Wellness

Preparing your own food is the only way to know what's in it, and when you're keeping track of what you're eating, you need to know exactly how much and what was used. For example, you'll want to know if your vegetables were sautéed or steamed. If they were sautéed, what kind of oil and how much was used? You can always ask your server, but they may not know or be misinformed.

When you cook your own food, you're in control, and home-cooked food tends to be better for you, too. I'll discuss different cooking methods and how some can make cooking faster, easier, and require fewer dishes to clean.

For someone who has never cooked before, it can be intimidating, but like any new skill, you need to educate yourself and practice to master it. I will share with you some cooking hacks to help you in the kitchen, whether you're brand new to cooking or a seasoned veteran.

Meal Planning Mastery

If you take a little time to plan out your meals, you can eat well and still have time to take care of your responsibilities and do the fun things that bring joy to your life and make it worth living. It's just like anything else; it may come naturally, or you may have to work at it, but planning and preparing your food in advance will take you to the next level of your health. If you are more of a "go with the flow" type, you can set yourself up for success by having healthy food options at home. Either way, make a grocery list in advance of going to the store so you're not tempted to buy unhealthy foods impulsively. Making time to meditate, exercise, visit with friends, and do self-care is important for overall health as well.

Portable Protein Solutions

Eating the right ratio of macronutrients can be challenging, especially if you lead a busy lifestyle, but it's possible if you're committed and prepared. I'm a planner and like to be prepared for whatever comes my way, so I try to have things ready when I need them, and I'm no different when it comes to food. When you look at the menu at most restaurants, the macronutrient ratios are usually off, and if you want to be successful, you'll need to make some slight modifications when eating out, and I'm here to help you with that.

Protein-heavy snacks are essential to have available between meals, so you're not forced to eat something you'd rather not. They're not as readily available as other snacks, but good options do exist, and I will tell you some of my favorites. I get irritable when I don't eat, so I always try to make sure I have some good snack options available wherever I go.

Let's Get Physical

If you want to live a long time, avoid injuries, and be resilient, you'll have to do more than just eat more protein.

You'll need to exercise and be physically active to keep your body strong.

Physical activity can be fun and can look very different from person to person; we all have different goals, body types, and activities we enjoy. I never enjoyed resistance training until a few years ago, but I really enjoy the challenge now.

Resistance training is not only great for building muscle; it also strengthens your bones and can help you lose a few extra pounds. Going for a walk every day could be enough for some, while others may need more. There are lots of options for improving your physical fitness, and the best part is that you can do a lot of them at home, like yoga, resistance bands, or simple bodyweight exercises.

A Holistic Approach: The Missing Piece

Having good mental health is vital to your success. If you don't care about yourself, you won't want to take care of yourself, and what is the point of all this hard work if you're not happy? You're in luck because there are lots of options when it comes to taking care of your mental health, or as I call it, "mental recovery." It could be simply making time to visit with friends, starting a meditation practice, talking to a therapist, or even practicing self-hypnosis.

Physical recovery is necessary, too. It can help with sore or tight muscles and flexibility. I have a lot of areas of my body that give me a hard time and cause me discomfort. I will share some proven techniques that I have used to reduce pain and inflammation and reduce the chances of injury in the future.

All the information I have and will share with you in this book is based on things I have learned over the years through trial and error or things I have researched and are backed by the scientific method. People have gotten weird about science lately. They claim this and that and say, "It's science." If you remember, back in middle school, you were taught about the scientific method and that experiments need to be repeatable to claim that something is proven science.

New food research, exercise methods, and how supplements affect us are being discovered all the time. One thing you can always count on in life is that things will change, and if you know that and are open-minded about new information, then you will always be ready for it. I'm excited to dive deep into all these topics with you in the upcoming chapters.

Are you ready to consider the information in this book and start applying it to your life to be your best self?

CHAPTER 4:
DECODING NUTRITION

In high school, I ate a bag of Flamin' Hot Cheetos and a Personal Pan Pizza with a side of nacho cheese most days for lunch. Deep down I knew this was not a healthy choice, but I didn't care. I was young and was not worried about my health. Now that I'm almost forty, I care a lot about my health because I want to have a good quality of life when I'm older and avoid as many diseases as I can by taking care of my body.

I never had a good relationship with food, and I still struggle to this day, but I try to do my best every day by eating the right balance of macronutrients to hit my goals, and that's what counts. To start eating better, you need to know how different foods affect your biology, and that is what will be covered in this chapter.

It's been a while since I took nutrition in high school, but I have done a lot of research on it since then. I'll get into the differences between macronutrients and micronutrients, discuss complete and incomplete proteins, the glycemic index, the gut microbiome, and the truth about cholesterol. I will also go over some tips and things to keep in mind when you're grocery shopping and how to set yourself up for success.

Macronutrients and Micronutrients

Macronutrients and micronutrients comprise everything we eat, and these terms are used to categorize the nutrients your body requires to operate. Macro means large scale, and this translates to the majority or bulk of the foods you eat. These include proteins, fats, and carbs. They are the main sources of fuel for your body. Micro means small and refers to things like vitamins and minerals that your body needs in smaller amounts. They support many bodily functions and overall health. You must consume the proper amounts of both to feel and look your best.

Macronutrients:

<u>Protein</u>

Protein is the most important macronutrient because it is the building block of tissues like muscle, bone, skin, and organs. It also provides amino acids that your body cannot make on its own and are necessary for proper nutrition.

The best source of protein is unprocessed, naturally raised organic meat from healthy and well-cared-for animals.

Protein is critical for:

- Building and repairing tissues
- Immune system function

- Hormone production

- Producing enzymes

<u>Fat</u>

Fat is the second-most important macronutrient. Your brain is pretty much made of the stuff, and it is an essential part of the membrane of every cell in your body. Fat also provides energy, is critical for the absorption of fat-soluble vitamins, and plays a key role in synthesizing sex hormones like testosterone and estrogen.

Some sources of healthy fats include:

- Coconut oil

- Red meat

- Nuts

- Seeds

- Avocados

- Salmon

<u>Carbs</u>

Carbs are the body's main source of energy but it is the only macronutrient that is not required for survival. However, carbs are an important part of a well-balanced diet. They get converted into glucose, and that's what fuels your brain and red blood cells. Carbs also get converted into glycogen, which gets stored in your muscles and is used during physical activities or during a fast.

Make sure you try to eat mostly whole grains and stick with organically grown foods to avoid glyphosate and other nasty chemicals. Fiber is also a carb; it can help keep you fuller for longer and slow down digestion to help avoid spikes in blood sugar levels. It also helps improve gut health and bowel movements.

Examples of healthy carbs include:

- Fruits

- Vegetables

- Whole grains

Micronutrients

Vitamins

Vitamins are essential for many processes in the body. They help with immune function, bone health, and energy production, to name a few. Most people are deficient and should supplement their vitamin intake with a daily multivitamin. The most efficient and scientific way to do this would be to get your blood work done regularly so you know the specific vitamins you are lacking, and then you can supplement those specific ones.

Good sources of vitamins include:

- Beef

- Fruits

- Vegetables

- Dairy products

<u>Minerals</u>

Minerals are vital for several bodily functions, like bone health and nerve and immune system functions. You could get all the minerals your body needs by simply eating *nose to tail*, which means eating every part of an animal, like the heart, liver, and brain. This can be hard for people like me who did not grow up eating these foods. Luckily, some companies make pills that contain freeze-dried and ground-up organ meats that you can take as supplements to get all the benefits of these organ meats without having to eat them directly.

If you can't stand the idea of organ meat, you could get your minerals from:

- Red meat

- Poultry

- Leafy greens

- Nuts

- Seeds

Essential Amino Acids

Proteins are made up of amino acids. It's vital to consume complete proteins or you will suffer from muscle weakness, have a slower recovery, and a compromised immune system. There are twenty types of amino acids, nine of which are essential. These are the ones our bodies cannot make on their own and need to be a part of our diet. When you have a protein source that has all nine of them, it's considered a complete protein.

Complete proteins are typically found in animal-based foods like:

- Chicken
- Beef
- Fish
- Eggs
- Dairy

Here are a few examples of plant-based complete proteins:

- Quinoa
- Amaranth
- Hemp Seeds

Incomplete proteins, however, are those that don't contain all the essential amino acids and are found in plant-based foods. Combining incomplete proteins like rice and beans makes it possible to obtain all the essential amino acids.

Some examples of incomplete proteins include:

- Lentils
- Nuts
- Seeds

It is important to note that if a significant portion of your protein comes from animal sources, you do not need to worry about incomplete proteins.

Gut Microbiome

One of the most important things to consider regarding nutrition is your gut microbiome. This is a community of microorganisms consisting of bacteria, yeast, fungi, and viruses that live in your intestinal tract. They help break down the foods you eat by consuming them and converting them into forms of nutrients your body can absorb.

Each type of organism feeds on specific types of food in your gut. These organisms will grow in number in proportion to the amount you eat. For example, sugar. When you eat more sugar, the population of sugar-eating organisms will grow, and consequently, you will crave it more. That is one reason why it's so hard to change what you eat, but the light at the end of the tunnel is that once you stop feeding them, they will die, and you will begin to crave those foods less.

Probiotics are beneficial gut organisms. To populate your gut with them, you should incorporate fermented foods in your diet.

Examples of fermented foods are:

- Yogurt

- Sauerkraut

- Kimchi

- Real pickles

Most pickles at the store are not fermented; they are pickled in a vinegar brine. You want to eat real pickles that have been fermented in a salt brine. Kombucha is a good option, too. Most cultures have at least one fermented food as part of their diet because these foods are so crucial for good health.

Thermic Effect

Have you heard of the thermic effect? It is not critical, but it is worth mentioning. The thermic effect or dietary-induced thermogenesis is the increase in calories burned due to the amount of energy required for digesting and processing the food you eat. When you eat food, your body uses energy to break it down, absorb nutrients, and transport those nutrients to various tissues in the body. This process requires energy and leads to an increase in metabolic rate; the rate at which you burn calories at rest.

The thermic effect varies depending on the type of food you eat, with protein having the highest thermic effect, followed by carbs and fats. In general, the thermic effect contributes to about 10 percent of most individuals total daily energy expenditure according to the Harvard School of Public Health.[3] In conclusion, if you eat more meat, you will burn more calories due to the thermic effect because your body will have to use more energy to break it down!

Glycemic Index

The glycemic index (GI) measures how quickly carbs raise blood sugar levels after they are consumed. This can be

---

[3] Harvard University. "Energy Balance: Totaling Up Energy Expenditure." 2023. https://www.hsph.harvard.edu/obesity-prevention-source/energy-balance/

helpful for anyone with diabetes, but the system is not perfect due to several reasons, one of which is that it changes when you combine different foods together. Foods with a high GI are digested and absorbed very fast, causing a spike in blood sugar that will lead to a crash, leaving you feeling lethargic and hungry shortly after consuming them.

In contrast, foods with a low GI are digested and absorbed more slowly, resulting in a slower increase in blood sugar levels, which will help sustain you between meals. Choosing foods with a lower GI can help support your overall health and fitness goals.

Some grains, for example, wheat and rice, are processed and stripped of fiber and nutrients to create white flour or white rice. It's better to stick with whole grains because they are lower on the glycemic index and have more nutrients. I always preferred jasmine rice as my grain of choice, but when I changed how I ate, I switched to whole-grain rice. It took a little getting used to, but it is delicious and nutritious.

Here are some examples of high and low GI foods:

High GI foods:

- Candy

- Cake

- Cookies

- White bread

- White rice

- Cornflakes

- Baked potato

- Watermelon

- Dates

- Pineapple

Low GI foods:

- Steel-cut oats

- Whole-grain bread

- Brown rice

- Sweet potato

- Apple

- Pear

- Broccoli

- Carrots

- Lentils

- Chickpeas

Foods low in carbs, like beef, chicken, fish, and other animal-based foods, generally do not have a GI value, but processed meat products, like sausages and deli meats, do contain small amounts of carbs from added sugars or other ingredients, which could impact their GI.

I grew up eating processed meats like sausages, hot dogs, and bacon, and I still enjoy eating them to this day, but I know I must limit how much I eat to maintain my health.

This is the difference between living and not *Living the Protein Lifestyle.*

You do not have to worry about GI if you are not diabetic and are only eating whole foods. This is due to the fiber content, natural sugars like fructose and glucose, and the additional nutrients found in whole foods.

Cholesterol

Remember the article I mentioned in Chapter 2 about how the Sugar Research Foundation sponsored a research program in the 1960s on heart disease? Well, they also blamed cholesterol, which is really messed up because it is a vital nutrient for many bodily functions, and a lot of people are still afraid of it. Plus, dietary cholesterol does not affect cholesterol levels in your blood. Cholesterol is used to form the building blocks for all the cell structures in your entire body and is critical for hormone production, digestion, and vitamin synthesis. It's also necessary to form brain cells and maintain healthy brain function. So make sure you are eating whole eggs once in a while, not just the whites; your brain will work better, and your breakfast will taste better, too.

Controversially, too much cholesterol can increase the risk of heart disease and stroke, making maintaining healthy cholesterol levels through a balanced diet and lifestyle modifications important. Your diet should include a balance of healthy fats like cholesterol.

Some examples of foods that contain cholesterol are:

- Fatty cuts of red meat
- Full-fat dairy products

- Shrimp

- Sardines

Whole Foods Versus Processed Foods

<u>Whole foods</u>

Whole foods are natural single-ingredient foods that come from the earth.

Whole foods are vastly superior to processed foods because they are rich in nutrients like vitamins, minerals, fiber, and antioxidants. The biggest differences are what is not in whole foods.

Some foods may look like whole foods but have been tampered with. Most people would never assume foods like precooked chicken bites would have canola oil (inflammatory), rice starch, or natural flavors (questionable chemicals).

One more thing you may not have considered about whole foods is their water content. Whole foods contain much more water than processed foods, and eating more whole foods will help if you have difficulty staying hydrated.

Examples of whole foods:

- Fresh meat

- Fruits

- Vegetables

- Nuts

- Seeds

Any of the foods listed above can become processed if they are not fresh, in their whole form, or pre-packaged. Make sure to check the labels. One rule of thumb is that if something is not in a package, it is most likely a whole food.

<u>Processed foods</u>

Processed foods are any foods that have been through some sort of process to make them taste better, last longer on the shelf, or look or smell better. There are even ultra-processed foods like breakfast cereals, fast food, and instant anything, including noodles.

Processed foods are designed to maximize profits for the companies that make them, using the cheapest ingredients. They also design these items to last as long as possible, so they remove all the nutrients because pests like mold feed on them.

Processed foods have been engineered to be hyper palatable and highly addictive. When these foods contain polyunsaturated fatty acids, also known as hydrogenated oils, they block your stomach's signals to the brain to tell you that you are full and to stop eating. One of the nutrients that's removed is fiber. That's how you can eat a whole bag of corn chips and not feel full.

Now, I can't have a chapter on nutrition and not discuss how to choose healthier options when shopping for groceries. One easy way to avoid chemical-ridden processed foods is to stick to the perimeter of the grocery store as much as possible. All the processed foods are typically in the middle aisles, while all the whole foods like fruits, vegetables, and meats are on the perimeter.

When you are shopping on the perimeter, there are no nutritional facts labels, so you'll have to do some research to determine the nutritional makeup of these items, but even if you do not take the time to do this research, you will naturally stop eating when you have had enough because these items are in their natural state with all their filling fiber or protein.

I've made it a habit to check most nutritional labels I come across. I like to know what the macronutrients are, how many calories per serving, the serving size, and most importantly, what it's really made of, as opposed to the marketing on the package. If you want to make more informed decisions, read those labels to educate yourself.

When shopping for food, the list of ingredients usually found under the nutritional fact label is one of the best tools to help you determine if it's a good food choice or not. The ingredients are listed in order from the most to the least by volume of each, so there will be more of the first item listed and less and less further down the list. This will help you gauge how much of a particular ingredient is in the product you're considering purchasing. If you see high-fructose corn syrup or vegetable oil near the top of the list, stay clear of that item.

One key takeaway for buying healthier food is that the fewer ingredients in a product, the healthier it probably is for you.

The rest of the nutritional facts label can help you know the micro and macronutrients contained within. The suggested serving size is also very important to your success. If you don't know how much a serving is, you won't be able to portion it properly and will likely overconsume it. Also, pay attention to how much protein, fiber, carbs, sodium, and sugar are in these foods. Now you know how important it is to balance these nutrients.

If you want to take your nutrition into your own hands, you need to know how to properly nourish your body to meet your health goals. Knowing the proper amount of each macronutrient and the total amount of calories you need to eat is how you get there, and the only way to do that is to use a macronutrient calculator. You can find one online or use the QR code below to check out the resource page on my website, to use the one I recommend.

joshnoland.com/resources

All you need to do is enter your age, sex, height, weight, amount of exercise you do, and your goal: to lose body fat, gain lean muscle, or maintain. The results will tell you how many calories you should eat and the amount of protein, fat, and carbs in grams you need to eat each day to hit your goal.

Then, you will need to track what you eat with a food-tracking app. The one I recommend can be found on the resources page of my website. Tracking what you eat can be tedious, but after you track for a while, you will get to know more or less the calorie and macronutrient content of the foods you eat, and eventually, you won't have to track anymore.

This can be overwhelming at first, but you will get the hang of it.

In the beginning, try focusing on staying within your recommended calories and, most importantly, eating the recommended amount of protein. This will keep you from overeating and keep you on track.

One of the main keys to long-lasting success is to not deprive yourself of any food, especially the foods you love or grew up eating, but to only allow yourself to eat them in moderation. You can always modify or replace these foods with better options, too.

For example, there is a baked version of Flamin' Hot Cheetos that has about half the fat and twice the protein as the original. I'm not recommending you eat either version due to the highly toxic and ultra-processed ingredients, but if you hit your macros and step count for the day, then you could reward yourself by eating a small amount of a preferred food. Eat it slowly and savor every bite to get the most out of it.

Rewarding yourself for accomplishing goals, however small they may be, is a great way to motivate yourself if you're struggling to get started. Keep in mind that rewards do not always have to be food; they could be any preferred activity.

Things you can do today to jump-start your transformation:

- Fill out a macronutrient calculator

- Download and start using a food-tracking app

- Start reading nutritional fact labels/lists of ingredients of foods you already have at home

- List five foods you love and how you could make them better for you

CHAPTER 5:
NOT ALL PROTEINS ARE CREATED EQUALLY

Are you opposed to eating meat? Are you wondering what high-quality protein actually is? These are great questions, and I will answer them in this chapter and reveal how all meat is not the same and that some ranchers care about the animals they raise.

There are many protein options: protein that comes from animals and protein from plants, but even those two categories can be broken down further. For example, beef raised and finished on grass can differ greatly from beef that is finished on corn and soy. All cows eat grass, but most are sent to feedlots to get fattened up before they are slaughtered. Grass-finished means no nasty feedlots. These lucky cows get to spend their last few months grazing on the pastures they were raised on. Plants can also differ in the way they are grown, harvested, and processed. This can greatly affect the quality of these plant foods.

Animal Protein

It's hard to imagine, but there is a big difference in the amino acid makeup of grass-finished beef. A cow that has only eaten grass its entire life has an equal amount of omega-3 and omega-6 amino acids, which is ideal for cardiovascular health. But cows fed corn can have up to a 10:1 variance in its amino acid makeup and, when consumed, contributes to plaque buildup in the arteries.

Biologically speaking, animal protein is the best source for your body regarding nutrient density and bioavailability. There are several factors you must keep in mind when sourcing these animal-based proteins. Meat from animals raised in natural environments is much healthier and of a higher quality than that from factory-farmed animals. Naturally raised animals are allowed to consume foods that they evolved to eat, which can provide a more diverse range of nutrients. They are also exposed to sunlight and fresh air, which contribute positively to the animal's overall health and quality of life.

Many people find that naturally raised meat tastes different. It has a more flavorful and richer taste than factory-farmed meats. This is because naturally raised animals tend to have a more varied diet and more nutrients, which can impact the taste and texture of their meat.

Factory-farmed animals are often given antibiotics and hormones to promote growth and prevent disease. This can lead to residues of these substances in the meat, which can have adverse health effects on us.

Naturally raised animals are often raised in a more humane manner as well. They are typically allowed to roam and graze in a natural environment, which can lead to less stress and better overall health.

Overall, meat from naturally raised animals is superior to meat from factory-farmed animals due to its higher nutrient content, better taste, and more humane production practices. Naturally raised meats can be more expensive and may not be as readily available, but if you look, you can find local producers. To reduce your cost, be prepared for shortages, and suport local ranchers whos practices you approve of, buy a chest freezer and purchase your meat in bulk.

Beef is one of my most preferred sources of protein. I love the flavor and the variety of things you can make with it. Beef is highly digestible, and its nutrients (amino acids, iron, zinc, and vitamin B12) are bioavailable. Plus, there are twenty-five grams of protein in three ounces of top round steak, so you don't need to eat a lot to get your protein fix. Some of my favorite beef dishes are slow-smoked Texas-style brisket, beef ribs, or filet mignon with salt and fresh cracked pepper.

Chicken is another great source of protein for several reasons: it's rich in high-quality protein, low in fat, and versatile as it can be prepared in many different ways, making it easy to include in a variety of dishes. This makes it easier to incorporate chicken into a healthy and balanced diet. One ounce of chicken breast contains around nine grams of protein.

Chicken eggs are an excellent option to get your animal protein because you don't have to kill the chicken to get them, and they can be used in so many different ways. You can boil, bake, scramble, or drink them raw if you're hardcore (I'm not). You could add them to ground beef to make a loaf or a hamburger patty.

Not all eggs are the same either, and it's hard to know what you're getting with all the creative labeling on the cartons, like cage-free, pasture-raised, organic—the list goes on and on. At the end of the day, eggs from chickens raised outside on pasture are usually of higher quality.

If you can keep chickens yourself, the eggs you would get from them could be some of the highest-quality protein you could get your hands on. I love chickens because they can recycle your food scraps and turn them into yummy eggs, and they are fun to have around. If keeping chickens is not an option, you can always try to find someone in your area who has them and try to buy eggs from them.

Now, let's talk about seafood. I love sushi and enjoy most types of seafood, but I'm not too fond of that fishy smell some fish have. Fish are good sources of protein and contain a good amount of vitamins and minerals. Fish is easily digested and absorbed as well.

Not all fish are the same, either. We have farm-raised and wild-caught, and these two can vary greatly in their nutritional profiles depending on their diet and environments. Farm-raised fish can be treated with antibiotics and are fed a diet of fishmeal, fish oil, and plant proteins like soy and corn. Fish would never eat plant proteins in the wild, and this can have negative health effects on them.

Some fish, like salmon and trout, are fed synthetic or processed feeds that enhance the color of their flesh so they look more appealing, but like us, these processed feeds are not good for the health of the fish, and we pay the price when we consume them. It's important that you eat organically raised fish to avoid any of these concerns. Wild-caught fish aren't given any antibiotics but may contain heavy metals or pollutants, depending on where they are caught. You have to do some research to find the best sources. For example, I like wild-caught Alaskan sockeye salmon.

Wild game is hands down the ultimate high-quality and most nutrient-dense protein. I grew up eating meat from the grocery store, which did not include meat from wild animals like deer, elk, or wild boar. It takes a little getting used to the taste because it's nothing like meat from domesticated animals that you buy at the grocery store. It could be described as gamey, earthy, tangy, or even nutty. Game meats are bold and full of flavor and take some getting used to. This is what meat is supposed to taste like. These flavors come from the variety of foods these animals eat, including additional vitamins and minerals from natural forage, which are lacking in domesticated animal meats.

I did some hunting with my uncle when I was younger and would like to do more in the future. It's a weird feeling eating something that you killed. It wasn't easy for me and may never be easy because I did not grow up hunting or ranching. Still, I realize the importance of knowing where your food comes from and helping to manage the population of these animals since we have killed off many of their natural predators. I hunt to put food on my table; well, it actually goes in the freezer, but you know what I mean.

Meat from game or wild animals is superior to all other meats because those animals eat a natural diet and live an organic lifestyle. This makes these animals very healthy and jam-packed with vitamins and nutrients that domesticated animals don't even come close to. I have to mention here that no one should ever hunt for sport because that is not cool. Even if you're killing animals for population control or because they are causing damage to crops, the meat from those animals should be used as a resource and not wasted.

It's also important to note that animal proteins differ in the amount of fat they contain. For example, salmon and sardines have more fat than cod or tilapia, while beef and pork have more fat than chicken and turkey. This is something to consider when planning your meals, as you do not want to overconsume fat, just like any other macronutrient.

Plant Protein

Now, let's discuss plant-based proteins. As you can probably tell by now, I am not a fan of getting protein primarily from plants, but I realize that there are people who just cannot eat meat for one reason or another, so here we go.

Unlike animal protein, plant protein is often lower in fats, so you need to make sure you are getting enough to ensure proper bodily functions. Plants are, however, rich in fiber, vitamins, and minerals, making them a good source of nutrients.

Plants cannot run away or defend themselves like animals. Instead, they use chemicals to discourage animals from eating them, and these chemicals can have negative side effects on your body when you eat them, so be careful to avoid plant foods you may be sensitive to.

I have noticed that there are more and more vegan and vegetarian food products available in the past few years that are highly processed, like Beyond Burger and chicken-less nuggets. These products are not good for you because there are lots of preservatives, hydrogenated oils, high fructose corn syrup, and other filler ingredients that are inflammatory and will have negative side effects if you overconsume them. Also, these processed foods tend to have less fiber and nutrients than their whole-food alternatives. If you choose to eat a vegan or vegetarian diet, I would highly recommend you eat as many unprocessed plant foods as possible.

Peas

Peas are a highly nutritious legume and are a good protein source. One cup of cooked peas contains approximately nine grams of protein. Peas are also rich in fiber, vitamins, and minerals, including vitamins C and K and potassium. Additionally, peas are low in fat and calories, making them a great addition to your diet.

The protein found in peas contain all nine essential amino acids, technically making it a complete protein, but it is low in one of these essential amino acids, so it should not be your main source of protein. Peas are processed and used as a base for many vegan food products, including protein shake powders, but they are most nutritious if unprocessed.

Soy

Unlike peas, soy does contain a good ratio of all the essential amino acids, making it an excellent source of protein. Like peas, soy is low in saturated fats like cholesterol and can be consumed in various forms.

Some people may not realize that soy is a bean and can be eaten in its whole form, known as edamame, a Japanese term referring to a young, immature soybean. They must be cooked well so they are more digestible; however, uncooked soy contains compounds that may interfere with nutrient absorption. Whole soybeans can be eaten by themselves with some salt, used in a salad, used to make a dip, or go into a soup.

Processed soy is used a lot in vegan and vegetarian diets and can come in the form of tofu, tempeh, milk, and many meat substitutes. Soy has been linked to several health benefits, including reducing cholesterol levels, lowering the risk of heart disease, and improving bone health.

However, it's important to be aware of the potential hormonal effects of consuming large amounts of soy because it contains phytoestrogens, a naturally occurring plant compound with a structure similar to the hormone estrogen. As a result, phytoestrogens can interact with the body's estrogen receptors and mimic some of the effects of estrogen. There is concern that consuming large amounts of soy may negatively affect fertility, hormone levels, and thyroid function in certain individuals. It's important to note that the research on the effects of phytoestrogens is still ongoing, and more studies are needed to fully understand their impact.

Overall, soy can be a healthy choice for incorporating additional protein into a plant-based diet, but I recommend you limit the amount you eat because it's in so many different products. You will see for yourself once you start looking at the list of ingredients on those nutritional fact labels.

Lentils

Lentils are another plant source of protein, they contain approximately eighteen grams of protein per cup of cooked lentils. They are also rich in dietary fiber, vitamins, and minerals such as iron, folate, potassium, and magnesium. They are low-fat and low-calorie foods and can be prepared in many ways, making them an easy and cost-effective way to incorporate more protein and essential nutrients into your diet.

A few more options for getting your protein from plants include:

Legumes: chickpeas, black beans, kidney beans, navy beans, pinto beans, lima beans, and peanuts (yes, peanuts are not true nuts; they are legumes).

> While legumes are a good source of protein and other essential nutrients, consuming too many can lead to digestive issues due to their high fiber content. The complex carbs in legumes can also cause bloating and gas in some people, particularly if they are not used to eating them regularly. One way to mitigate this is to soak your legumes in water for an hour or two prior to cooking them.

Nuts: almonds, walnuts, cashews, pecans, and pistachios.

> Nuts are a good source of protein because they contain healthy fats and fiber. Be careful not to eat too many because nuts are very calorie-dense. The serving size for pistachios with the shell is about half a cup. I like to get them with the shells, so it takes me

longer to eat them. Nuts are portable and will last a while in your pantry. For a healthy dessert, I like to make chocolate-covered pecans or almonds. All you need to do is melt some dark chocolate in the microwave and use it to coat the nuts. Spread them out on a plate and then throw them in the freezer for fifteen minutes to harden the chocolate.

Seeds: pumpkin, chia, sunflower, hemp, and sesame.

Seeds have healthy fats and other important nutrients like iron and magnesium. I enjoy snacking on roasted and lightly salted pumpkin seeds; they are a good source of protein and fiber, and they help cure my cravings for salty foods. When you eat them one at a time, a one-ounce serving can last you a while when you are watching a TV show or a movie. Also, hemp seeds are another one of the rare whole protein sources that come from plants.

Grains: Quinoa, amaranth, rice, oats, corn, and couscous.

The grains listed above have a higher protein content than most other grains, but it is still relatively low. You would have to eat a whole cup of sweet corn to get only 4.7 grams of protein. Grains are also high in calories and can easily be overconsumed.

Vegetables: Spinach, broccoli, peas, Brussels sprouts, and artichokes.

Like grains, vegetables are not a good source of protein because they simply do not have enough of it. They do have a lot of fiber and other important nutrients like vitamins and minerals, and that's why it is important to eat them.

Nutritional yeast is a deactivated yeast commonly used as a seasoning in vegan and vegetarian dishes that provides a nutty and cheesy flavor to foods. Nutritional yeast is a good source of protein—at five grams per tablespoon—and vitamin B12, making it an important ingredient for people who may have difficulty obtaining sufficient amounts of vitamin B12 from plant-based sources alone. It can also add an extra layer of flavor to various dishes.

Spirulina is a blue-green algae cultivated and harvested for its nutritional benefits and is commonly sold as a dietary supplement. Spirulina is a good source of protein, vitamins, and minerals and has been associated with various health benefits, such as reducing inflammation and improving blood lipid levels. One tablespoon of dried spirulina has four grams of protein.

As I mentioned at the beginning of this chapter, not all proteins are created equally, and I choose animal protein as my preferred protein source because it is superior to plant protein in many ways. If you just can't eat animal protein for whatever reason, ensure you are getting enough high-quality protein, essential amino acids, and B12.

No matter where you get your protein, make sure you get enough of it, and the rest will all fall into place. The goal is start slow and do the best you can with what you have. This will propel you forward to better health.

As you explore the world of protein sources, what will you choose to put on your plate?

CHAPTER 6:
YOU CANNOT CHANGE WHAT YOU DO NOT MEASURE

So you want to improve your health but hate dieting? Me too! I don't like having to follow a strict diet and not being able to eat the foods I enjoy.

Back in 2019, when I started taking my health into my own hands by exercising and making better food choices, I started changing my diet by tracking the amount of calories I was eating. This was a good start, but I did not see a significant change in how I looked and felt until I started paying attention to the macronutrients. I had to start gradually, but with time, I was able to adjust my meals so they fell within the recommended ratios for my goals.

Back then, my goal was to lose body fat. That means eating more protein to mitigate the amount of muscle mass I lost and to be in a calorie deficit. In English, that means to consume less calories than I burned each day, so my body would be forced to burn fat to make up the difference.

Early on, I struggled with eating too many fats due to the fact that I love eating red meat, dairy, and fried foods. As I mentioned before, dietary fat does not necessarily corelate to body fat, but it is high in calories and should not be overconsumed. I mentioned my struggle to my wife, and she told me "You need to isolate your fats." I did not know what that meant. She explained. "You need to cut out fats where you can so you have more control over how you eat. For example, try low-fat dairy products or remove the yolk from your eggs." This made sense to me, and once I started doing just that, I was able to reduce the amount of fat I was eating and stay within my macros.

In school, your teacher would track your progress and give you a letter grade to let you know how you were doing. That was how you knew if you needed to study more or not. The same principle goes for nutrition, but you will have to take on the role your teacher once did. When you first start eating for better health, the only way to know if you need to adjust the amount or type of food you eat is to remember everything you eat, how many calories it contains, and the macronutrient breakdown. More realistically, you will have to keep track with a food log app in the beginning. Making sure you eat the right amount of calories to hit your goal is a good start, but you'll need to track more than that to achieve success.

Keeping a paper food journal is okay, but it is a lot of work to manually input all the information. It's much easier and less time-consuming to use an app that will fill in the calories and macros for you.

As with most new things, I recommend you start slow by logging what you are already eating. Once you have a few days logged, go back and see how your current diet compares to what's recommended by the macronutrient calculator. This is when you can gradually start adjusting what you eat until you're within the recommended amounts of calories, proteins, fats, and carbs per day.

Yes, you can have ice cream, but you need to read the nutritional facts label to ensure you know how much one serving is and how many calories, protein, fat, and carbs are in that one serving. If you adjust what you eat around special snacks or rewards, then you don't have to deprive yourself of anything; you will have to plan it out and make good choices.

I love drinking Coke and have since I was a child. I know it has a lot of sugar, and I should try to avoid it. There is Diet Coke, but it just does not taste the same, and it has artificial sweeteners, which I also try to limit. What a dilemma! I have decided for now to allow myself to drink up to one mini can of Coke a day as a reward for hitting my daily step goals.

The most important macronutrient to track will, of course, be protein. Make sure to eat the protein portion of your meal first. Doing this will ensure that you get your protein in for one, but you will also not have as much room in your stomach to overconsume carbs because the protein that is so satiating will make you feel full.

Pro tip: Eat your higher-protein snacks first, too.

If you start significantly increasing your meat consumption, the next most important metric to track will be fiber. Fiber helps keep you feeling full and helps with digestion. You may need to bump up the amount of fiber you are getting because eating a lot of meat without enough fiber could make you constipated. Ask me how I know! Your food tracking app will tell you how much fiber you need.

Some high-fiber foods I enjoy include:

- Avocados (10 grams per medium-sized avocado)

- Raspberries (8 grams per cup)

- Blackberries (6.7 grams per cup)

- Chia seeds (5 grams per tablespoon)

Sample day of tracking my food intake:

Breakfast	Calories	Carbs	Fat	Protein
Stacked Peanut Butter Protein Shake	315	25	4	50
Egg, Egg Whites, and Cottage Cheese	183	3	6	25
	498	28	10	75
Lunch				
Deep Dish Pizza, Pepperoni, 2 Slices	693	80	28	32
Canned Chicken Breast	210	0	4	46
	903	80	32	78
Dinner				
Grass Fed Filet Mignon, 5 oz.	188	0	8	29
Persian Cucumber, 2 each	36	8	0	0
	224	8	8	29
Snacks				
Nonfat Plain Greek Yogurt, 1 cup	133	8	0	24
Blueberries, 1 cup	42	11	0	1
beef jerky, 1 oz.	90	0	3	16
Organic Popcorn, 3 cups	100	19	1	3
	365	38	4	44
Totals:	1,990	154	54	226
Daily Goal:	2,234	223	50	223
Remaining:	244	69	-4	-3
	Calories	Carbs	Fat	Protein

Accurately tracking your food intake is important for reaching your health goals. I recommend you start out by weighing your food because that is the most accurate and precise way to figure out how much of each item you're consuming. I bought a small digital scale that I kept with me to weigh my food when I first started tracking my food intake seriously. After doing it for a few months, I knew more or less how much something weighed and didn't have to use the scale as much. I suggest you use a scale when you start because if you're off a few ounces here and there, it makes a big impact on your totals for the day, and that could be the difference between you getting to have that extra snack or not and ultimately achieving your goals.

I want you to be able to have that extra snack and feel good about it. Earn it by staying active and eating well throughout the day. This is another example of rewarding yourself—a trick I use all the time to help me do all kinds of things.

Here are some tips I have used to successfully track my food intake:

If you're having difficulties staying within your limits, don't be super-critical of the amount of calories you consume daily but try to focus on your total intake for the week. It's not super-important to hit your numbers every day, but eating the right amount over time is important and will help you if you are not consistent.

Tracking can get tedious, but it can also be fun. Try making a game out of it. See how many days in a row you can track, and if you do it for a week, reward yourself by eating a preferred food or doing something fun.

The best practice is to enter what you're eating just before, during, or just after you eat it. It's easy to forget what and how much you ate or get busy and forget to log altogether. I tend to log my food as I'm eating it.

Another way to find long-term success and not feel restricted in what you eat is to plan what you're going to eat in advance. You can log the foods you most want to eat for that day and then fill in the rest to hit your macro and calorie goals. For example, if you want pizza for dinner, enter that in your food tracker in the morning and then fill in the rest. You may want to include a salad or some veggies with dinner to balance out the meal, and if you need more protein, try adding some canned chicken breasts to your salad or on top of your pizza.

You can save a ton of time by saving your recipes in the app MyFitnessPal for things you cook regularly. I have my daily protein shake and a few other staple recipes I use almost every week saved in the app. It's easy. All you have to do is create a new recipe, add the ingredients, select the serving size, and save it. Then, when you need to log it, you select it from the list and add it to your food diary.

If you subscribe to the paid version of MyFitnessPal, you can scan bar codes of food items and log them in very quickly and accurately. I only encountered a handful of items that were not already in the system when I scanned the barcode. There is also a new option that will let you take a picture of your food, and it automatically detects the food item and calculates the portion size. I have not tried it and do not know how accurate this new feature is.

One last tip for accuracy in logging what you eat is to look for items that have been verified. You will know they have been when you see a green badge with a checkmark next to the item. Some entries are way off, so I recommend double-checking them against the nutritional facts label occasionally. This is where being diligent will really help you get an accurate picture of your nutrition.

You can start right now! Download a free food-tracking app and log everything you eat today.

If you consistently track what you eat for thirty days, it will become a habit. After a few months or a year, you will better understand the macronutrient makeup of foods and won't need to rely on an app anymore.

Being mindful of what you eat can be hard sometimes, but it will have a huge impact on how you feel physically and emotionally. It's so easy to self-soothe after a hard day by binge-eating, but it's not worth it in the end. Instead, go for a walk or meditate to relax, and then go make yourself a high-protein, low-calorie dessert.

If you track what you eat and stay within some basic guidelines, you can eat anything you want in moderation. You will have to pick and choose what you allow yourself to eat, but nothing is off-limits. This is the way. I mean, this is how you live the protein lifestyle.

CHAPTER 7:
HOME COOKING: A RECIPE FOR WELLNESS

I enjoy cooking but I love eating!

Eating good food is one of the many joys in life. By good food, I mean, flavorful food made with love that nourishes my body and soul. It is hard to quantify how food made with love is better but there is just something special about food made by someone who cares about the people they are cooking for, even if it's only for themselves.

There are many benefits to cooking your own food. You get to choose the ingredients you use and how much, making it easier to track what you're eating more accurately. Choosing the ingredients you use can be particularly important if you have any food sensitivities or foods you want to avoid. You can also get more food for your money and serve yourself the correct ratio of macros.

Like I said, I enjoy cooking, but cleaning up afterward can be annoying. But if you clean as you go and utilize certain cooking methods, it can make cleaning up faster and easier. Cleaning as you go could include using the same measuring spoon or cup and rinsing it off in between uses or planning the preparation and cooking of your meal in such a way as to use less equipment. Grilling tends to be less messy than cooking on your stovetop, and following one-pot recipes will reduce the number of dishes that need to be washed.

Do whatever you can to make cooking at home more enjoyable, whether that includes involving your loved ones or playing music. Whatever you choose, make it fun!

I went to culinary school for a year, and one of the best things they taught me that I loved and still use is a French term called *mise en place*. This translates to "everything in its place." This means before you start cooking, you have everything needed to make the dish—washed, chopped, measured, and ready to go.

Have you ever started cooking and, halfway through, you realized you forgot to prepare something? Chopping onions, for example. You have things cooking, and then they start to get overdone or even burn because you have to stop and try to quickly chop some onions, and it all goes downhill. I have, and it sucks the joy right out of the whole experience. I have been known to get overwhelmed in the kitchen once in a while, and having everything ready to go helps me feel like I have everything under control. This idea of prepping everything beforehand makes cooking more enjoyable and ensures you have everything you need to get the job done.

Try it next time you make food at home and see if this method works for you. It could make the difference in finding success in the kitchen.

Cooking Oils

Do you know what kind of cooking oil they use at your favorite restaurant? Most restaurants use cheap vegetable or seed oils that can cause inflammation and block the signals from your stomach to your brain that let you know you are full and to stop eating.

Lipids are a group of molecules that are insoluble in water, also known as fats and oils. You can tell if something is an oil because it is liquid at room temperature, whereas fats are solid at room temperature, but the terms are mostly interchangeable when it comes to cooking.

Animal fats from naturally raised animals are some of the best to cook with because they contain important vitamins, have a high smoke point, add rich flavors, and keep you feeling full. People have been using them for thousands of years and have thrived.

Only in the last one hundred or so years since we started using highly processed seed and vegetable oils have we seen such a rise in obesity and many other health-related issues. I'm not saying this is solely due to cooking with these industrial oils, but I don't think it's a coincidence either.

The Good:

I prefer animal fats like tallow, butter, and lard because they taste great, are packed with nutrients, and are a valuable resource from the butchering process. It's also part of eating nose to tail.

It's important to note that fat is where toxins are stored, so make sure to get your animal fats from naturally raised animals that were not given growth hormones or antibiotics.

I also enjoy and recommend these minimally processed plant-based oils:

- Olive

- Coconut

- Avocado

The oils above can be produced via a cold-pressing process and do not require complicated procedures or harsh chemicals, thus producing a more natural and healthier product.

The Bad and the Ugly:

Highly processed refined vegetable oils to avoid:

- Soybean oil

- Canola oil

- Corn oil

- Cottonseed oil

- Sunflower oil

- Safflower oil

- Peanut oil

- Sesame oil

Have you seen how these oils are made? Solvents, bleach, and other harsh chemicals are used in an industrial process to make these oils. I try to avoid consuming them as much as possible, and I advise you to do the same.

These oils are commonly used in processed foods, fast food, and traditional restaurants due to their affordability, availability, and high smoke points. However, these oils have an unhealthy balance of omega-3 and omega-6 fatty acids. In the past, we used oils with a 1:1 ratio of these fatty acids, but these vegetable oils have a 20:1 ratio of omega-6 relative to omega-3. Scientists hypothesize that eating a diet high in these oils may lead to chronic inflammation, and chronic inflammation is an underlying factor in heart disease, cancer, diabetes, and arthritis.[4]

Additionally, consuming too much of any type of lipid can lead to weight gain and other health problems, so it's important to use them in moderation as part of a balanced diet.

Cooking Methods

Let's discuss some cooking methods for all these high protein meals you're going to start preparing at home now that you know how important it is to choose the right foods and prepare them the right way. There are tons of cooking methods, from grilling to sous vide and lots in-between, so you have a lot of options.

---

[4] Kris Gunnars. "Are Vegetable and Seed Oils Bad for Your Health?" *Healthline.* Updated June 9, 2023.
https://www.healthline.com/nutrition/are-vegetable-and-seed-oils-bad

<u>Pressure Cookers:</u>

Recently, one of my go-tos is the pressure cooker. You can make a good volume of food in a relatively short amount of time. There's less to clean, and you can automate it to some extent. You can even cook meat that's frozen in a pressure cooker if you're in a pinch.

I use an instant pot because it's so versatile. You can sear a piece of meat, sauté your onions and garlic, deglaze with some red wine, and then throw the meat back in and pressure cook it until it's fall-apart tender—all in one pot. That's four different cooking methods using one pot. Imagine the time you will save when doing the dishes.

Pressure cookers are good for cooking all kinds of one-pot meals, like pot roasts and all kinds of soups. I really like them for cooking chuck roasts. This is a tough cut of beef, and by pressure cooking it, you save time compared to using a slow cooker, and the meat gets just as tender, juicy, and full of whatever flavors you choose to impart to it. For example, you can make birria, teriyaki beef, beef and broccoli, or, my favorite, a simple braised beef that can be served in a variety of ways.

<u>Grilling:</u>

I enjoy and recommend grilling to anyone who loves the outdoors and the smell of meat cooking over an open flame. Whether it's propane, charcoal, or wood-fired, there is just something so special and primal about it. I love grilling year-round. How badass is it to cook a steak on your grill in the snow? I have done a few times when I lived in the mountains.

When I cook a filet mignon on the grill, I like to keep it simple. I'll add coarse salt and fresh cracked pepper, and then all it needs is about three to five minutes on each side for a perfectly cooked medium-rare steak—oh my, it's heavenly.

Some people have a favorite style of grilling. In my case, it depends on the situation. If you're hungry, tired, and low on time, a propane grill can be a great option. They're easy to light, get to a cooking temperature quickly, and you won't reek of smoke too much after you're done cooking. It will give your food a slight smoky flavor without all the hassle of dealing with hot coals or ash when you're done.

If you have more time, you can use a charcoal or wood-fired grill. If you want a bit more smoke flavor imparted in your food, use charcoal. Charcoal is made from wood that's burned in the absence of oxygen. This process removes the water and volatile compounds, leaving you with almost pure carbon. Charcoal burns very hot and has minimal smoke.

If you're looking for more smoke flavor, you can cook with wood. Initially, it won't be as hot as charcoal and will give off more smoke, but once the wood burns down, you are left with coals, similar to cooking with charcoal.

Smoking meat is different from grilling, but I wanted to mention it here because I enjoy the art of smoking meats, and it has some similarities to grilling, like cooking outside and using wood and charcoal as fuel. If you like a lot of smoke flavor and have all day, try smoking some meat in an offset smoker. My personal favorite is a smoked brisket or poor man's burnt ends made with a chuck roast.

You can change the flavor profile of the foods you grill by using different types of wood and, subsequently, charcoal. Mesquite is used in southern and Tex-Mex dishes and is described as having a bold, smoky flavor that is slightly sweet and earthy. Some of the best grilled chicken tacos I have ever had were grilled with mesquite. Oak is a great choice for a milder smoke flavor that won't overpower the flavor of the meat. Ultimately, the type of wood you use comes down to personal preference and availability.

<u>Cast Iron:</u>

Then there is the old reliable: the cast-iron skillet. Cast iron is great because it has no toxic chemicals like nonstick pans, retains heat well, imparts iron into your food, and can last for generations if cared for properly.

You can use a cast-iron skillet to cook almost anything. Sauté, roast, broil, or braise—it can do all those things and more. If I could only have one pan in my kitchen, it would be a twelve-inch cast-iron skillet. Cast iron can take many forms, such as Dutch ovens, griddles, grates for grills, and even woks. Dutch ovens are great for camping or at home; you can bake bread, make cobblers, or braise meats in them.

There are a few tricks to working with cast iron.

For one, don't clean it with soap, or you'll remove the nonstick polymerized layer, also known as the seasoning. If you're having trouble with food sticking and need to reseason your cast-iron cookware, all you have to do is apply a thin coat of oil and bake it in the oven at 400 degrees for twenty minutes.

To properly clean your cast iron, clean it while it's still hot. This will make the job a lot easier. Pour out the fat, and then use hot water and a metal sponge to scrub off any stuck bits. If the bits are really stuck, you can use coarse salt to help scrub them off. Once it's clean, you need to dry it thoroughly to avoid rust. You can do this by putting it back on the stove for a few minutes to evaporate all the water. Then, apply a thin coat of oil all over the pan to protect it.

Carbon steel is similar to cast iron in the way you clean and care for it, and it won't leach chemicals into your food. It's thinner than cast iron, so it heats up faster and does not retain heat as much, making it easier to adjust your cooking temperature on the stove to avoid overcooking your food.

Sourcing High-Quality Ingredients

If you want to take your health into your own hands by cooking your own food, you need to use the best ingredients possible. Depending on your financial situation, this could look very different. In the best-case scenario, you'll want to use fresh organic produce, naturally raised grass-finished beef, pasture-raised chicken and pork, and wild-caught fish. If you can grow your own, that would be the best, but you may not have the time, knowledge, or space to do so. If you can't afford the best of the best, it's okay. Sticking with whole foods that you prepare is a much better option than processed, fast food, or even most restaurants. You don't always need to eat at home, but the more you do, the better your health will be.

No matter where you live, you can always find a way to get the whole food ingredients you need to make food that tastes good and properly nourishes your body. Whether you use a food subscription box, buy directly from local producers, or shop at farmers' markets, you will find a way to make it happen.

Buying food in bulk is a good way to save money, and unless you have a large family, you will have to store it. You have a few options, like canning or freezing, but you will have to figure out what works best for your situation.

When I was in my twenties, I ran my own cooking classes. I would instruct the class as we prepared a meal, and then we would all sit down together and eat it. It was a lot of fun, and I learned a lot from my students and guest chefs.

I have been developing and perfecting my own protein-centric and health-focused recipes for the past fifteen years, and I'm very excited to share a few with you. Use the QR code below, to get my top three high-protein, easy-to-make recipes to kick-start your health journey delivered straight to your email inbox. I will also be releasing a cookbook with tons of delicious recipes that will help you hit your macros and nourish your body, so keep an eye out.

proteinlifestylecookbook.com

Cooking at home is a valuable skill to have, and knowing exactly what you are eating will go a long way toward improving your health and quality of life. If you have zero cooking experience, now is the best time to start learning. There are so many videos and recipes online that you won't have any trouble finding some guidance. I used to love watching a TV show called *Good Eats* with Alton Brown. He would break down the science behind cooking, and I enjoyed learning the hows and whys of cooking.

I learned a lot from that show. One of the most important things was to be empowered by cooking and making it your own. If you don't have a certain ingredient, don't worry about it; substitute it for something else. The worst thing you can do is give up because you're missing one ingredient. For example, if you're making chicken soup and you don't have parsley, don't worry about it—your soup will still taste great. You should customize recipes to your tastes and goals anyways. If you don't like an ingredient, swap it for something else or omit it altogether. If a recipe calls for soy sauce and you want to avoid soy, use coconut aminos.

One of the best things about cooking your own food is that you can make it however you want. Use recipes as guides, not strict rules you must follow exactly unless you're baking. That is more of a science than an art, and you need to follow the ratios, times, and temperatures for the end product to come out right.

My dad had his own catering company since I was three years old, and he started it out of our house, so cooking was always a part of my life. I started helping my dad in the kitchen when I was five. We would make our own pizzas together, and my love of cooking grew from there. Cooking with others can be fun and a great bonding experience. If you have kids, teach them to cook when they are young, and they will be set for life. We have to eat food every day to live, and if you know how to cook, then you do not have to rely on others and can be more independent.

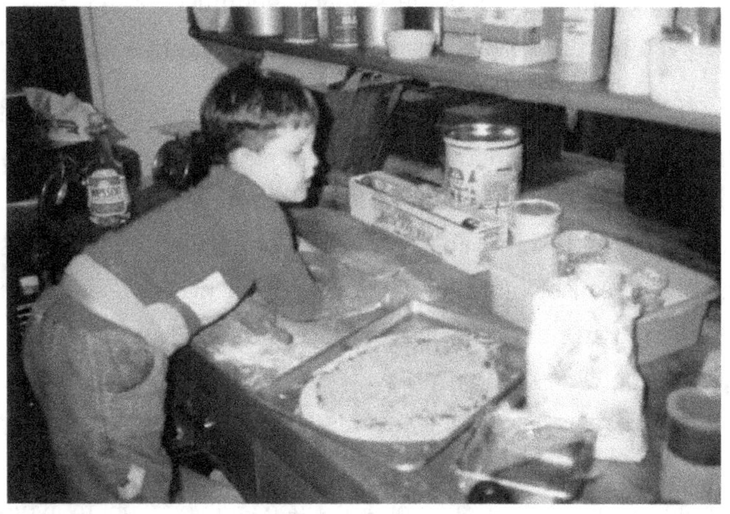

The author making pizza with his dad when he was five years old.

Since I started changing my eating habits for my health and subsequently cooking more of my own food, I have been able to consistently eat the right amount of protein, fat, and carbs and mostly avoid the highly processed foods that are having such a negative impact on our health today.

I encourage you to try cooking more at home to help you take control of the food you eat, and put your health in your own hands. If you need help, you can always reach out to the *Living the Protein Lifestyle* Facebook group (QR Code below), and if you don't need help, you can always share pictures of the dishes you make or find inspiration or ideas.

facebook.com/groups/livingtheproteinlifestyle

When was the last time you cooked dinner at home? Try it tonight and start *Living the Protein Lifestyle*!

CHAPTER 8:
MEAL PLANNING MASTERY

Have you ever wondered how those gigantic cargo ships are able to sail across the vast expanse of the ocean and arrive at a specific port at a designated time and day despite encountering stormy weather and treacherous currents? Along the way, the crew must make critical decisions and adjust their course as necessary to navigate the hazards and reach their goal.

The key to a successful journey is that there is a clear destination. Without a destination, the ship would be adrift and directionless, at the mercy of the winds and waves. But with a goal to aim for, the crew has a sense of purpose and direction, which helps them to stay motivated and focused, even when faced with obstacles.

Having a clear idea of what you want can help you navigate the challenges and uncertainties you will encounter. By having something to aim for, you can stay motivated, make better decisions, and overcome any obstacles that might otherwise derail you.

In this chapter, I offer how, when you take the time to plan out your meals and prepare food in advance, you are much likelier to be successful at eating healthier. I'll also share with you some of the strategies I used to find success in navigating a world full of fast and convenient unhealthy foods.

One way to set yourself up for success is to make it easier to make good food choices. The easier it is, the less likely you'll be to ditch your goals when things get tough. Once you find a few well-balanced meals that you enjoy eating, you can start incorporating them into your regular diet and then add in new ones to keep it novel.

Planning out your meals a week at a time is ideal, but if that's too overwhelming, you can start out by planning your meals one day at a time. You have to start somewhere, and taking the slow and steady route is better than wandering aimlessly and succumbing to unhealthy temptations. If your schedule is consistent from week to week, it will be easy to incorporate meal planning into your regular routine.

If your schedule is more inconsistent, then you may need to be more active in ongoing meal planning. Don't worry if you don't have a regular routine. I got you. Change is the one constant in life, and knowing that will go a long way. Plus, I'll share some of the tips I use for getting my protein on the go in the next chapter.

Meal planning is simply deciding in advance what you are going to eat, and with the valuable information you're learning in this book, you will have a good idea of what foods and how much of them you should eat. When you sit down to plan, you have some options. You can use a note app, a notebook, or a calorie-tracking application. The key is to plan out what you want to eat to hit your nutrition goals and have it ready when you need it.

Batch Cooking

One way to save time is to cook in bulk, also known as batch cooking. When you cook a large amount of food in one go, you save time by not having to cook and clean up after every meal. This works especially well for lunches. Whether you are at work or not, at lunchtime, it's nice to be able to eat a healthy homemade lunch without having to interrupt your day by taking the time to cook a whole meal and deal with all the dishes.

Batch cooking does not have to include cooking: it can be combining several items together to make it faster to prepare something for later, like a protein shake. When I want my post-workout protein shake, I don't want to waste time. I just want to drink it and get on with my day. That's why I make up several batches at once, and this is how.

I start with several containers laid out on the kitchen counter. Then I'll add protein powder to each container, peanut butter powder, creatine powder, and so on until I have added all the dried components. Then, when I'm ready to drink a shake, all I have to do is dump the dry ingredients in my blender bottle, add my liquid of choice, shake, and chug it down. Quick and easy. That's how you find success in achieving your goals: by making it easy and convenient.

Chuck Roast

I really like boneless chuck roast because it's economical and so versatile in how many different dishes you can make with it. Whether it's pot-roast, teriyaki, shredded beef birria, or barbacoa, these dishes are delicious and quick to cook when you use a pressure cooker like an instant pot.

I like to cook a two and a half to five-pound chuck roast, eat some fresh, and then freeze the rest in individual portions. It's convenient to have these preportioned ready-to-eat foods in the freezer because you can defrost them as you need them, they last a long time, and they thaw quickly.

Here is my method. Once the meat is cooked, I'll let it cool to room temperature and then divide it into six-ounce portions. You may want to use different portion sizes depending on your macronutrient requirements or if you're preparing food for others in addition to yourself. Once the meat is weighed and placed in separate containers, I evenly distribute the cooking juices among each container. Keeping the cooking juices in the container will keep your meat moist and add more flavor when you reheat it.

Chicken Breast

Grilled, baked, or pressure-cooked chicken breast prepared in bulk to use throughout the week is another great option. This will save time and take your meal planning to another level. Lightly season it so you can use it in a variety of dishes. I use a little salt and fresh cracked black pepper. Once you know how you will be using it, you can add more seasoning or sauces to enhance the flavor.

Chicken breast can be used to top off a green salad, make a chicken salad, in tacos, or by itself as a very protein-dense snack. There are a lot of options.

When I cook chicken breast in bulk, I plan it out so I can eat some fresh, and then once the rest cools down, I slice it, store it in four-ounce portions, and keep it in the refrigerator.

<u>Boiled Eggs</u>

Eggs are a great source of protein, and when you hard-boil them, they can be a great snack or used for many different recipes. You can make a bunch at a time and keep them in the refrigerator for several days.

I like to use them to make a low-fat, high-protein egg salad by replacing the mayonnaise with cottage cheese and removing the yolks from several of the eggs. You could also make deviled eggs, chop them up and add them to a salad, or eat them as is.

A few more items you can cook in bulk to use throughout the week:

- Seasoned ground beef, turkey, or chicken

- Breakfast burritos

- Brown rice

- Beans

- Lentils

Preparing a lot of food at a time will save you time throughout the week by reducing the overall food preparation, cooking, and number of dishes you have to clean. Even the most dedicated health enthusiasts eventually get tired of eating the same thing every day, so make sure to be on the lookout continuously for new recipes, so you can cook a variety of meals.

Batch cooking is a key strategy I use for meal planning, and it also works well for those weeks when I have too much going on to plan out all my meals. When there are healthy and delicious foods in my refrigerator or freezer that are pre-made and ready to eat, I am less likely to eat out and make poor food choices.

Meal Planning Methods

I utilize a few different methods for planning my meals. Sometimes, I'll use Evernote, a note-taking application I use every day for all kinds of different notes to help me stay organized, like writing this book. If you're new to tracking calories and macros, the best way to ensure that the meals you're planning meet your nutrition requirements is to use a food-tracking app. Lastly, if you live with someone else who wants to be involved in the process, you can use a dry-erase board for meal planning. This way, everyone can see it and be part of the process. You could also use all three of these methods if you're a freak like me.

Note-Taking Application

When I use a note-taking application like Evernote to plan out my meals, I start by writing out each day of the week and each meal, including snacks for each day. Once you do this for the first time, you can reuse the note as a template, so you don't need to write out the days and meals every week.

Now that I have my template, I'll start adding the most important macro for each meal, which is, of course, protein!

I do this in the kitchen while I'm taking proportioned meats or raw meat that I buy in bulk like from my Butcher Box delivery out of the freezer to defrost and use for the week. These proteins are the foundation of most of my meals, and if I need more, I'll add them to my grocery list.

Once I have all the proteins accounted for, I'll look to see what else I have on hand that will pair well with the meat and make complete meals. I'll then proceed to add those items to the note. Now, all I have to do is fill in the gaps and add whatever is missing to my grocery list.

If I'm not going to be home for any of the meals, I will indicate that on the note and plan how to accomplish my eating goal wherever I may be.

Food-Tracking Application

When I want to be really precise in planning my meals, I'll use a food tracking app like MyFitnessPal to log everything I want to eat for a day so I can see exactly how much of each item I should consume and where my macronutrients and calories will be coming from. From there, I can adjust my plan by adding or removing different food items to see how they affect the numbers.

I recommend you try this when you're first starting out so you can learn the proper portion sizes and the nutrient makeup of the foods you eat. Once you do this for a while, you will know how much and what you need to eat to nourish your body and reach your goals.

<u>Dry-Erase Board</u>

If you are planning meals with others or if you are someone who needs visual reminders, using a dry-erase board to plan out your meals could be a good option. You can use the same procedure as the note-taking application for this method.

Whatever method you use for planning your meals, find something that works for you and stick with it, and if it stops working, try something else. It takes some planning to get the right amount of macros you need each day to be healthy and strong, but it's worth it.

As I write this, I am in a cutting phase. This means that I'm trying to reduce body fat and minimize the amount of muscle I lose. This is achieved by reducing calories and increasing protein. Don't worry. A macronutrient calculator will figure this out for you. As you can see above, my daily protein goal is 223, and that is a lot, but with some careful planning, I was able to get very close to my daily goals. I did go over a little on protein and fat, but not by much, and I was slightly under in calories and carbs. This is ideal and will average out over the week.

It might not be easy at first, but you will get there. I definitely don't eat like this every day, but it's my goal to keep trying and that's what's most important—that you keep trying and don't give up. Just because you messed up one meal or one day or even a whole week, all that matters is that you get back on course and keep trying.

HOW TO INCREASE YOUR PROTEIN INTAKE

Eggs

Adding eggs to your meal to bump up your protein is great, but be mindful of the fat. Eggs are packed full of nutrition, and you can prepare them in so many ways, but if you eat a lot of them, you'll need to remove some of the yolks to reduce the fat, unless you're in a bulking phase but even then it could be too much. Fried sunny-side up, scrambled, poached, boiled, or baked in a frittata, eggs are great for you, easy to cook, and so versatile! Unless you are allergic, you should be eating eggs.

If you are sensitive to corn or soy, look for corn- and soy-free eggs. They may be hard to find, but they're out there. They may not trigger a negative reaction like eggs that come from chickens that are fed a diet high in corn- and soy-based feed. If you just can't seem to find them or you want the most nutrient-dense eggs ever, get some chickens and make your own. It's not too much work to keep a few chickens around if you have the space—you can get away with having just a few hens in most places.

Meat-centered meals

Eggs are a good way to add protein to a meal that needs a little extra, but if you make the protein the base of the meal, then you will be ahead of the game. Decide on a whole protein and how much you need to hit your per-meal macro goal, and then figure out the rest.

Greek Yogurt

If you get an unflavored nonfat Greek yogurt, it could have as much as eighteen grams of protein per three-quarters of a cup. If you add protein powder, then it could really bump it up.

Okay. Here it is. The easiest and most effective piece of advice in the whole book. Are you ready? If you want to successfully live the protein lifestyle, all you have to do is eat your protein serving first whenever you eat. Before you eat any carbs or fats, eat your eggs, Greek yogurt, or drink a protein shake. When you do this, you ensure you are going to consume all your protein, which is required for building muscle, and more muscle makes you stronger and more resilient so you can avoid injuries and diseases. Now if you are feeling full and don't finish all your food, it's okay because you've already got the most important macronutrient taken care of. This goes for snacking, too, so eat that beef jerky before you go snack on some popcorn.

Side note: I love popcorn, but I don't feel bad eating it when I make it at home with a reasonable amount of salt and a healthy oil like coconut oil. It tastes so good and is easy to make; you should try it.

Here are a few examples of how to get fifty grams of protein in one meal or snack:

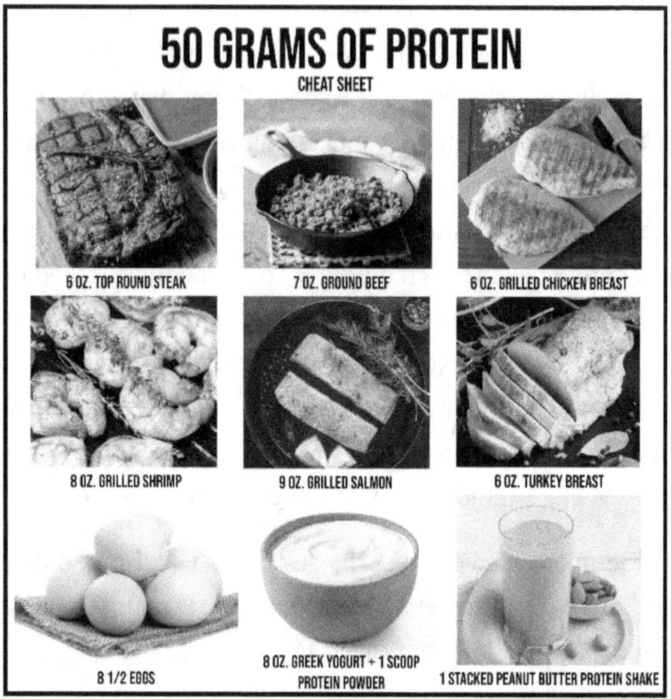

Meal prep tips to help you save time in the kitchen:

These options may not be the highest-quality foods, but they are better options and more convenient. If you make things too hard, you will be more likely to quit. We are looking for progress, not perfection.

Pre-Chopped Salads

I'm not a big fan of prepackaged food, but it's important to get some greens in your diet for the added fiber. It takes time to do all the washing and chopping, and if you have a lot going on like me, you may not have time. You may live alone or be the only salad eater, and it doesn't make sense to buy all the fixings to make a salad because it may go bad before you can finish it all. Pre-chopped salads may be a better option for you because they come with everything you need and tend to be only a few portions, so you can eat it all before it gets all slimy.

Bonus tip: If you hold back on the dressing and use less than the suggested serving size, you drastically cut down on the calories and fat, and if you pair your salad with your protein of choice, you can make it a very well-rounded part of your meal.

Rotisserie Chicken

A rotisserie chicken from the grocery store is an inexpensive and fast way to get a precooked whole protein that you can use in a lot of ways. The chickens they use are not free-range, but it's better than getting fast food.

When I get a rotisserie chicken, I'll start by peeling off the skin and throwing it in the air fryer until it gets crispy and golden brown. Now you have something I like to call chicken chicharron. The smell of fried chicken and the crunchiness mixed with the fat and salt—it's absolutely to die for.

While the chicharron is cooking, I'll take the breast meat off the bone and set it aside. This can be eaten as is, on a sandwich, or used to make chicken salad, chicken dip, or as a salad topping.

Then I move to the leg quarters, which include the leg

and thigh, and I remove them from the rest of the carcass and set them aside. Sometimes, I'll debone it to make tacos or eat it with rice. Or just eat it off the bone.

Now, I pick the rest of the meat off and save it for later. You can use the bones to make broth or soup if you like. Just drop it in a pot of water with carrots, celery, and onions. Let this boil for an hour or more if you want bone broth—strain and enjoy.

This parted-out chicken will last in the fridge for several days, so you don't have to use it all right away. One of my favorite things to do with chicken is to make a buffalo dip or quesadillas.

Concentrated Broth Bases

There are many different options on the market for condensed broth bases made of cooked meat and/or vegetables that can be used in a variety of ways. You can find beef, chicken, and vegetable bases that help with making a simple soup or adding flavor to your favorite meal. They are a really fast and easy way to add tons of flavor to your dishes. I use the beef broth base as the cooking liquid when I make my chuck roast, which is so flavorful. I have used the chicken broth in steamed rice, and I've also drank the broth straight up when I had a sore throat or a cold, and it really helped me feel better. I use and recommend the Better Than Bouillon line of concentrated broth bases.

Frozen Herb Cubes

Any little thing to help make cooking at home easier is great because the fewer barriers you face, the more likely you will be to succeed, and cooking at home is the best way to know exactly what you're eating. These frozen herb cubes make adding flavor to your dishes as simple as popping out a cube or two and get cookin'. You can skip the washing and chopping.

Can you tell that washing and chopping are not preferred activities of mine? The cubes are equal to one teaspoon and come in garlic, ginger, and basil. The better your food tastes, the higher the chances you'll actually eat it, and the less prep you have to do will make you want to cook at home more often!

Freezing Precooked Portioned Meats

I touched on this already but wanted to go into more detail here since I have had a lot of success using this method. By cooking a lot of meat at a time and then freezing it in separate proportioned amounts, you can reduce the amount of detail that goes into meal planning. If you're not meal planning, this method works great too because you can use these proteins immediately if needed by defrosting them in the microwave, and depending on what it is, you can finish heating it in an air fryer or in a sauté pan.

One last word of advice on this: make what you're freezing as flat or thin as you can; it will freeze faster and take up less room, and on the flip side, it will defrost much quicker.

When I hurt my back and recovered by getting more active and losing weight, I did not plan my meals and was not able to keep the weight off. I was missing the nutrition component of my health plan. But in 2019, when I started working out and was mindful of what kind and how much food I was eating, I was planning my meals and knew how important it was to eat right. I really believe that was a big part of my long-term success.

Planning out every meal may not be right for you, and that's okay; it's not for everyone. Honestly, sometimes I get tired of it, or I get busy with life. As long as you have good food options available, you'll find success.

Have you tried meal planning? Try it for a week. Even if you're a seasoned planner, try using some of the techniques I have offered, see how it goes, and let us know in the Facebook group.

Make those critical food decisions in advance and adjust your course as needed to reach your nutrition goals, and you will do great!

CHAPTER 9:
PORTABLE PROTEIN SOLUTIONS

Our modern-day lifestyle seems to keep us on the go and doesn't seem to leave a lot of time to plan and prepare for much of anything, let alone our meals and snacks. Even if we find the time to make a plan for what to eat, it does not always go as intended. We need to consider what to do in these situations before we get there. When I get really hungry, it's like a primitive part of my brain takes over and doesn't care about my daily macro goals; it just wants FOOD.

Have you ever been getting ready to go somewhere, and you're kind of hungry but not ready to eat yet? You say to yourself, "I'll just grab something on the way." Most of the time, when this happens, you have good intentions, but then you get hungry, and your intentions fall out the window. Now you're starving, and you stop at the first drive-through you see and get whatever looks good.

I know because this happens to me every once in a while, but I try my best to avoid it by being prepared so this part of my brain doesn't get a chance to take control. I always try to have good snack options with me or a plan to find them wherever I go.

One of my go-tos is pumpkin seeds. One ounce of pumpkin seeds has over 9 grams of protein, 2.3 grams of fiber, and only 176 calories, and they can easily fit in your pocket.

Set yourself up for success when you're getting ready for your day by packing some snacks in case you get hungry in between meals.

Here are some on-the-go snack options to consider:

<u>Beef Jerky</u>

Beef jerky is a great option when you're on the go. It's very portable and high in protein. Make sure to find a brand that doesn't have too much sugar; most brands have a lot. Beef jerky is processed meat, but we are looking for better alternatives. Remember, progress not perfection.

If you don't like beef jerky, they make turkey and pork jerky too. I like People's Choice original beef jerky. It has zero sugar, tastes great, and one ounce has 18 grams of protein.

Biltong is similar to beef jerky but is traditionally less processed and made without sugar. It originated in South Africa and is made with beef or game meats. They marinate the meat in a mixture of vinegar and spices and then let it air dry. I have seen it available in some stores here in the US, and you can make it at home. It is a great alternative to beef jerky and a protein-rich snack.

Egg Bites

Egg bites are tasty and widely available. You can get them hot and ready to eat at Starbucks or buy them at Costco and Sam's Club. They are delicious, nutritious, and semi-portable as they need to be refrigerated, but these little snacks pack a big punch, coming in on average at twenty grams of protein for two of them. You can make them at home, too. They are made with eggs and cottage cheese as the base. Then, you can add protein, cheese, or vegetables to customize them. A great tip to make for an easier clean-up is to bake them in silicone cupcake liners. You can use steak, chicken, or whatever you like; get creative. I haven't tried it, but I bet brisket egg bites would be the bomb! Whether store-bought or homemade, these have been a go-to for me since they are so convenient. Pop them in the microwave for a minute, and you have a yummy, protein-rich snack!

Protein Snack Packs

P3 protein packs are one brand of protein-centric snacks that contain one portion of each of the following: meat, cheese, and nuts. For example, turkey, cheddar cheese, and cashew clusters. I really like that one because the clusters have dark chocolate on them, and it's a nice little treat. They are not very expensive and they're convenient and I have seen them sold at most grocery stores. I would not rely on these too much because these are processed meats and they are not the best for you, but they're better than candy and other junkie-type foods.

High-Protein Yogurt

If you're not sensitive to dairy, then high-protein yogurt is a good option. I really like the Oikos triple zero vanilla Greek yogurt. It tastes good, has fifteen grams of protein per serving, zero added sugar, zero artificial sweeteners, and zero fat. Plus, they come in a convenient single-serving size, which is convenient to grab and go. I have tried the other flavors Oikos has and do not like them as much because they leave my mouth feeling dry.

There are other brands of high-protein yogurts, like Too Good, a brand I recently learned about from a friend. They taste good and have twelve grams of protein and only two grams of sugar.

You can also make your own high-protein yogurt by adding protein powder to nonfat Greek yogurt. I like to do this in the evenings as a dessert. Sometimes, I'll add in some peanut butter powder and dark chocolate chips for a special treat.

Here is my portable protein solutions cheat sheet:

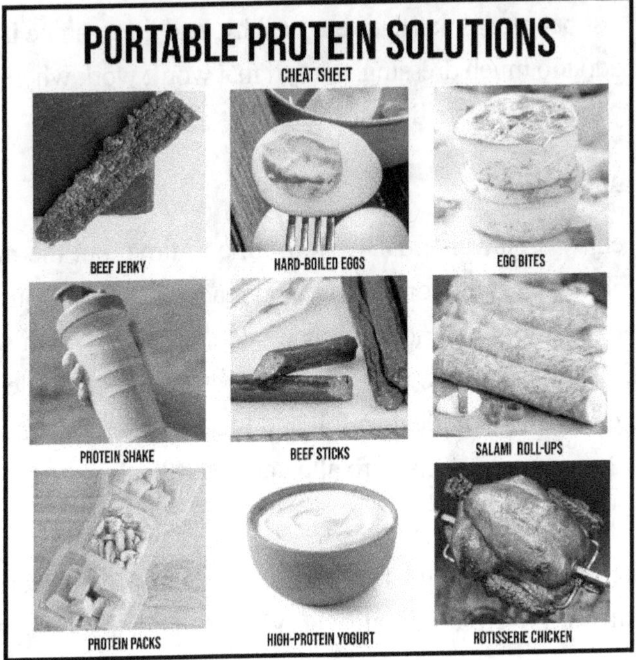

Making better choices when dining out

Eating at a restaurant when you're conscious of the types of foods you are eating can be difficult, but if you have a plan or at least some go-tos in your back pocket, you'll be able to stick to your eating goals. So keep these next few recommendations in your back pocket for the next time you're going out for dinner.

If you're at a steak house, you'll have a lot of grilled meats to choose from; just be wary of those side dishes. Lots of them are very carb-heavy. Try to get some sort of grilled or roasted vegetable or a side salad. Make sure to get the dressing on the side so you can use an appropriate amount. It's good to be in control of how much salad dressing you use because it is high in fat. Most people think salads are healthy, and they can be if you don't add too much dressing. Alas, if that won't work where you are, try some of these ideas instead:

Hawaiian BBQ

I enjoy a Hawaiian BBQ from time to time, but the meals are carb-heavy in the form of rice and macaroni salad. Don't get me wrong. I love the rice and mac salad, especially with some sriracha hot sauce: the one with the rooster on the bottle. All those carbs make me feel so full and tired after I eat them, plus they exhaust most of my carb allowance for the day.

I love the chicken katsu. If you're not familiar it's chicken thigh pounded flat and dredged in a panko crumb mixture and fried. I only allow myself to have this on special occasions since I limit the amount of fried food I eat. But when you dip that shit in the katsu sauce and take a bite of that crunchy panko breading, then taste the sweetness of the sauce mixed with the salty savoriness, it's pure bliss. Sorry about that. I'll get back to my point now.

Here's what I do so I can still enjoy some Hawaiian-style BBQ and stay on track. If I'm going for straight-up protein, I'll order two sides of either barbecue beef or chicken or one of each. This is a good portion, and it's more economical than a combo meal.

If I want some carbs, I'll get a mini meal or a kid's meal plus an extra side of meat. The mini meals come with one scoop of rice, as opposed to a regular combination meal that comes with two scoops and one scoop of macaroni salad. This is still a lot of carbs, but if I plan the rest of my day accordingly, I can still stay under my daily carb goals.

<u>Olive Garden</u>

It's extra challenging to make good choices at certain restaurants, like Olive Garden, where the majority of the dishes are pasta-heavy, but you can do it if you put your mind to it. I'm not a huge fan of Olive Garden, but it has a lot of options for the whole family, so I find myself there once in a while. When I'm there, I'll order a protein á la carte, like grilled chicken parmigiana with a side of broccoli, and if I want to treat myself, I'll order the nongrilled chicken parmigiana with a side of broccoli, and I might even have a breadstick.

I usually just try to eat just one breadstick, but they are just so tempting when they are right there on the table. If you have poor willpower (we all do at times), ask your server to bring only bring a few breadsticks.

Here are a few more examples of better options at places like Olive Garden:

- Side of meatballs

- Side of grilled chicken breast

- Sirloin steak

- Grilled salmon

<u>Fast Food Chinese</u>

Fast service-style Chinese food can be a good option if you know what to get. Panda Express is everywhere on the

West Coast, where I grew up, and the food is good (all things considered), and the macros can be on point as well. When I go to Panda Express, I like to get the "plate." It comes with a side and two entrées. When I'm sticking to my plan for the sides, I get half fried rice and half super greens, and for the entrée, I get a double portion of the grilled teriyaki chicken. This meal does have a lot of fat, but it does have a lot of protein, a reasonable amount of carbs, and a little fiber.

Most restaurants in the US serve hamburgers, and eating hamburgers with extra patties is a good option in a pinch. Make sure not to get extra cheese because the patties already have a high-fat content.

As I have mentioned previously, eggs are a good option to add protein to meals, and when you're eating on the run, it's no different. A lot of restaurants serve eggs, and you have a few options on how they are prepared, so you can mix it up.

If you find yourself at an eatery and you don't know what you should get, start by scanning the menu for all the protein options, disregarding the fried ones, and then start picking out a few that work for you. Then, pick a side that will help you hit your macros, like a salad (dressing on the side), fresh fruit, or vegetables. A lot of people have food allergies and sensitivities now, so waiters are used to custom orders. Just be polite, and you should not have an issue. If you're at a place that doesn't take custom orders, just order the best option and try your hardest not to eat the things that will make you miss your mark.

If you have the option of choosing where to go, don't make it hard on yourself. Go to a restaurant with lots of protein options, like a steak house or a barbecue joint, or just go to In-N-Out and get a 2x3. *"What is that?"* you ask. It's two slices of cheese and three patties, and make sure to skip the fries and the soda and save those animal-style fries solely for special occasions.

Additional protein is also available in unexpected products like Black Rifle Coffee Company's ready-to-drink espresso mocha. This eleven-ounce coffee drink tastes great, supports veterans, has 200 milligrams of caffeine and seven grams of protein per can.

There are lots of ways to get that little extra bit of protein, whether you're at home or on the go, and every gram is critical for you to be able to achieve your daily goal.

The other day, I was running late to meet up with an old friend, and I didn't get a chance to eat before I left the house or take a snack with me. I was hungry, and as you know, this is where we can get into trouble. The first place I saw was Taco Bell. I know, I know! Like I said, I was already hungry, so I went to the drive-through and got a chicken quesadilla and a crunchy taco combination meal with a Pepsi and a cheesy gordita crunch. Obviously, this was way too much food and not a good choice.

If I had only taken a moment to grab some beef jerky or anything small to hold me over, I would have been able to make a better choice. When I got home that day, I put a mini beef stick and a small pack of trail mix in my backpack so I have some options next time I'm running late and need something to munch on until I can choose something to eat that will help me feel good and increase my health.

Regardless of what establishment you choose to visit to satiate your hunger, try to make better choices when you can, and you will find success. You can do this!

CHAPTER 10:
LET'S GET PHYSICAL

In an effort to maximize your health, you must consider a holistic approach. Eating a proper diet is a critical factor, but moving your body and staying active are just as important. Mental health and wellness are part of it, too, but I'll go deeper into that in the next chapter. Strength training, cardiovascular training, and mobility are the topics that will be covered in this chapter.

Before I started working out back in 2019, I was angry and depressed a lot and could come off as short or uncaring. I was not happy with my lifestyle or how I felt, and I would constantly obsess about all the problems of the world, like the negative impact we have on the environment and all the problems with the food and medical systems. It would make me angry to think of those things on top of dealing with everyday issues at work and home.

When I started working out and going on hikes, I noticed that I didn't feel as angry because I had an outlet for those emotions. I would use all that negativity to fuel my exercises and push through my sets. This helped me feel better, be nicer, have more patience, and get stronger all at the same time. I also believe that going out in nature was very beneficial for my mental health.

Even though the problems I mentioned just a couple of paragraphs ago still exist, I don't obsess about them or let them affect me like they did because I'm in a better place mentally. I do what I can and don't let things that are out of my control consume me.

Eating a proper diet alone is not enough to keep your body functioning in optimal condition. You need to use your muscles to keep them strong and do mobility exercises to stay flexible to avoid injuries and have a high quality of life. A lot of people seem to see fitness as a chore or work, but exercising can be fun and rewarding if you do it right.

Many people nowadays work in an office and/or live a sedentary lifestyle outside work or school, and it's easy with social media and the endless amount of TV shows and movies available to stream. It's hard to get people to get off the couch, but it's so important to move your body regularly. Recently, I heard somewhere that sitting is the new smoking. This may be controversial, but sitting for the majority of your day is detrimental to your health, and if you want to live a long and healthy life, you should try to do more and sit less.

It may be challenging to start exercising. One way to make it easier is to use a pre-workout. These are pre-made drinks or powders you mix with water that taste good and give you a huge boost of energy. They usually have caffeine to increase energy and alertness. Beta-alanine for endurance and reduced muscle fatigue. And a whole lot of other hard-to-pronounce ingredients.

Be careful not to overdo it, as these pre-workouts can be intense. Like most of my advice, I recommend you take it slow and start with a small amount to see how it affects you. Also, be mindful not to become reliant on pre-workout drinks. Take a break once in a while. Look for brands that list all the ingredients as opposed to ones that say "Proprietary blend," so you know all that is in it. I also look for ones with no dyes or sugar.

Honestly, you don't need pre-workouts, gym memberships, or anything else to get started. All you have to do is get up and start doing something. The motivation and endorphins will come if you put in the work, and you will feel better about yourself.

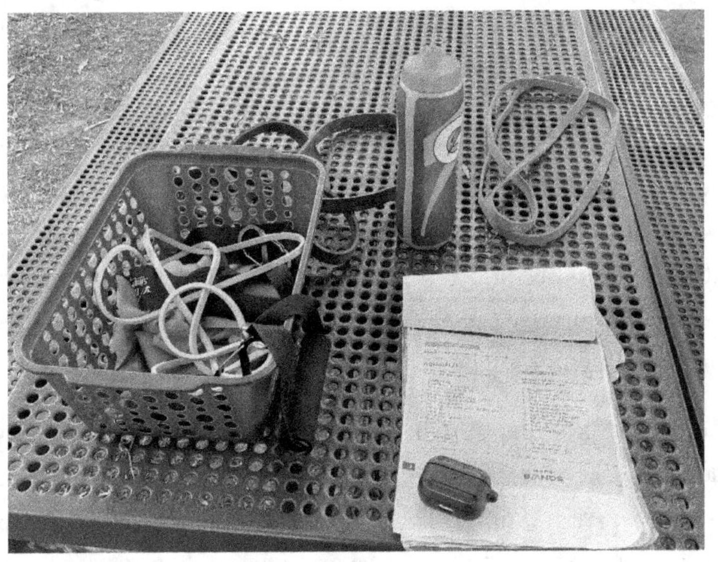

The author's basic home gym setup.

<u>Strength Training</u>

Strength training is one of the most health-promoting activities we can do. Whether you're lifting weights or doing body-weight exercises, it will promote muscle growth and strengthen your bones.

This is especially critical the older we get, so no matter what age or stage in life you're at, you should be doing some form of strength training regularly. You can join a fancy gym, use resistance bands at home, or get a job where you move heavy things around. No matter how you do it, just do it, and as long as you don't overdo it, your health will benefit.

You may be worried about looking too muscular if you start working out, but in reality, it's not that easy. It takes lots of hard work, dedication, and hours in the gym every day to get ripped like Dwayne "the Rock" Johnson. "Can you smell what I'm cooking?" That's a little saying the Rock used to say back in his pro wrestling days.

If you have never worked out before or it's been a while, take it easy and start slowly. You don't want to hurt yourself. Make sure to stretch, warm up prior to workouts, and pay attention to your body. If something hurts, stop what you're doing and modify the exercise to overcome any weaknesses or injuries you may have.

Resistance bands can be a great option because they don't take up a lot of space, and you can bring them with you when you're traveling. I used them extensively when I was on a two-month-long road trip and was able to work all my muscle groups and stay in shape on the road.

On the days that I do strength training, I focus on three main areas of my body: upper, lower, and core. I try to do compound movements that work more than one muscle at a time, like squats and push-ups. These movements help me to be more coordinated and have functional strength. Functional strength simply means being able to do things like squat down to pick something up or get up off the floor easily after playing with the dogs.

Examples of strength training:

- Weight lifting

- Bodyweight exercises

- Resistance bands

- Yoga

- Isometric training

Cardiovascular Training

When I hurt my back in my teens and the pain management meds and physical therapy didn't work, I decided to start swimming every day. This helped heal the bulging discs in my back by increasing my core strength without putting pressure on my spine. Swimming is a wonderful full-body activity that can be fun and refreshing on a hot day, and the low-impact nature allows you to get a cardiovascular (cardio) workout without putting a lot of stress on your joints.

Cardio workouts are important to keep your heart strong, improve blood flow, increase lung capacity, and increase stamina and endurance. It is not particularly good for weight loss as the body adapts to it quickly by slowing down your metabolism to conserve energy. That is why I only do it once a week and focus primarily on strength and mobility.

One key difference between cardio and strength training is the frequency. Cardio is low intensity for a longer duration, whereas strength training is high intensity for short durations, with rest periods in between sets to allow your heart rate to slow down. This is because these exercises focus on two different energy systems in the body: aerobic and anaerobic. Aerobic uses oxygen, and anaerobic uses glycogen stored inside your muscles.

Examples of cardio exercises:

- Running

- Bike riding

- Swimming

- Dancing

Mobility

Mobility is often overlooked, but it is important for flexibility, avoiding injury, posture, blood circulation, joint health, and healing from injuries to muscles, ligaments, and tendons. It can help you have a better range of motion, for example, bending further to reach something on the floor or reducing the likelihood of injury due to muscle strains.

Mobility is mostly stretching and body movements. It's like putting oil in your car engine; it helps to keep your joints lubricated and functioning properly. It also helps loosen up your muscles and keep you limber. Doing mobility exercises improves stability, therefore reducing the chance of a falling injury. These movements also release endorphins, which make you feel good.

Examples of mobility exercises:

- Shoulder dislocates

- Quad stretch

- Wrist circles

- Downward dog

- Lunge with a twist

I have weak joints and can easily hurt my knees, elbows, shoulders, or wrists by not stretching, so I make sure to do it as much as possible. My favorite form of mobility is yoga. Yoga classes combine meditation, strength training, and stretching. There is nothing more rewarding than completing a hot yoga class. You sweat buckets, but if you make it out alive, you feel empowered and ready to take on anything the day has to throw at you.

My Fitness Routine

Most days, I wake up around 5 or 6 a.m. and get myself ready for the day. Then I feed our dogs Hercules, Max, and Turbo and prepare for our morning walk. This achieves a few goals. I get early morning sun to help my circadian rhythm (helps me wake up and sync my internal clock), I get fresh air and time to think about things, and I get a jump-start on my step goal for the day.

When we get back from our walk, I make a pre-workout (not every day) and start with some stretching and warm-up movements. After I'm warmed up, I'll start my workout for the day.

Here is my workout schedule:

Monday: Strength training

Tuesday: Mobility exercises

Wednesday: Strength training

Thursday: Mobility exercises

Friday: Strength training

Saturday: Cardiovascular exercise

Sunday: Self-Care

After my workout, I'll do some cooldown movements and some more stretching.

Within an hour of my workout, I drink a protein shake to help start repairing and rebuilding my muscles. It's important to consume protein within a few hours of exercise to maximize your hard work.

As far as breakfast goes, I usually participate in intermittent fasting to help me stay on a calorie deficit because I'm in a cutting phase (reducing body fat) by not eating first thing in the morning. I let my digestive system fully digest what I ate the previous day. This helps reduce stress and inflammation in the gut. I also enjoy working out on an empty stomach, so it works out well.

I'll go about the rest of my day and then go for another walk after dinner. In addition to my exercise routine, I also have a daily step goal of 10,000–20,000 steps.

This routine allows my muscles to rest in between strength training days and gives me one day to really get my heart going to keep my cardiovascular system functioning properly. The mobility days allow me to be more flexible and have an increased range of motion. Take a rest day to let your body repair and rebuild. Your body needs rest to properly repair and rebuild.

<u>Step Goal</u>

Walking is a fantastic way to stay active: it provides many benefits, is free, and is good for the environment (if you walk somewhere rather than drive). Walking is a low-impact way to stay active and has been shown to increase cognitive functions like creativity and memory. It can be a social thing or done alone to give you time to think and ponder the meaning of life.

Find a friend or a dog to go on a walk with if you don't want to go alone. I love how fresh the air feels on early morning or evening walks, and I enjoy listening to the birds sing. Going for walks after eating speeds up your metabolism and helps with digestion, too. You have a lot of options; you could go for a hike in the woods, explore your neighborhood, park at the far end of the parking lot, or take the stairs. Either way, get outside, enjoy some fresh air, get some sunlight on your skin (for vitamin D production), and move your body.

I recommend trying to get in at least ten thousand steps every day as a minimum. Most cell phones have a built-in step counter, so you can keep track. You may not want to go for a walk, but you can't wait until you feel motivated. You have to make yourself, and once you do, you'll feel proud of yourself and hopefully continue going for walks daily.

Pro tip: Time your walks around the nicest parts of the day or walk inside a mall or the equivalent if it's just too hot, like Phoenix, Arizona, in the summer, or too cold, like Helena, Montana, in the winter.

You don't have to go to the gym or lift weights, but you should be moving your body daily, or you will suffer negative health consequences, both mental and physical.

There are many ways to stay active, from taking your dog for a walk to joining your local pickleball pickup game. I remember swimming at my grandparents' pool in the summers growing up and really enjoying that. I still enjoy swimming to this day, and it burns lots of calories.

Sports are a fun way to stay active and meet people at the same time. I loved playing dodgeball as an adult. I joined a league for a few years in Los Angeles when I was in my late twenties. It was so much fun to see everyone and play together once a week. It motivated me to eat better and work out so I could play dodgeball better. There are adult softball leagues or pickup basketball games too.

Having a team of smart and educated people to turn to when you have questions, are unsure of what direction to go in, or need inspiration is critical for success. I find it much easier to get motivated when I listen to podcasts or watch videos about fitness and health.

I have some of the resources I rely on located on my website's resources page. Check them out for help getting motivated or finding specific answers to your questions or problems you may face. Hopefully, I have or will answer many of those questions in this book, but I will not be able to cover everything, nor do I claim to know everything.

A friend of mine once told me that the human body is made up of over 70 percent water. Do you know what happens to water when it stands still for too long? It goes stagnant, starts developing detrimental microorganisms, and becomes unhealthy. That's similar to what happens to the human body when you don't move. So get up and start moving more if you want to feel good and have a higher quality of life!

CHAPTER 11:
A HOLISTIC APPROACH: THE MISSING PIECE

The last piece of the protein lifestyle puzzle is recovery. This can be broken down into two areas of focus: mental and physical. Mental recovery is about mindset and doing things to improve your mood and reduce stress and anxiety. Physical recovery is about doing things to help your body recover from stress, whether this stress is from exercise, work, or play. Taking care of yourself mentally and physically is just as important as what you eat and do. There is a lot of overlap in these areas. For instance, things you do to help with your physical state can affect your mental state and vice versa.

<u>Self-Care Sundays</u>

About a year ago, I started a ritual called Self-Care Sundays. Every Sunday, I take time to do something for myself. Usually, I do a face mask. I like the clay masks, but

I also do the paper masks once in a while. I know it looks weird and may not be for everyone, but I feel that it's important to take care of yourself, and your face is what people see the most, so I try to keep it at optimal health.

This self-care ritual doesn't have to involve face masks; it could be a foot or hand mask. Seriously though, it could be going to buy that pair of shoes you should have bought last month because the pair you're wearing hurt your feet or getting a manicure. Whatever it is, I try to do something for myself on Sundays, and I would suggest you try to do something like this, too, especially if you take care of others in your life and don't focus on yourself much. A small thing like this can make a big impact on your self-worth and might motivate you to do more for yourself like working out or eating better.

<u>Challenge</u>

Completing challenging tasks will leave you with a feeling of accomplishment. This feeling can put you in a positive mindset, which is the whole point. I'm saying you should test yourself by doing mentally and physically challenging things, like completing a difficult hike, a long bike ride, twenty minutes in a sauna, or three minutes in a cold plunge. These are great ways to boost your mood and self-confidence.

Doing things that challenge your mind is critical for brain health. Your brain is like a muscle in the sense that if you don't use it, you lose it. The more you work and challenge your brain, the stronger it will be. Try downloading and playing some brain games, do a crossword puzzle, or play chess. Whatever you decide, make it fun, and give your brain a workout at least once a day to keep your mind sharp.

<u>Sleep</u>

Sleep is the biggest factor to overall health and well-being.

Not only is getting enough sleep important but getting quality sleep matters just as much. Experts like Andrew Huberman recommend getting seven to nine hours of quality sleep each night for optimal functionality. Getting the proper amount of rest affects your mood, immune system, and energy levels throughout the day.

When you sleep, your brain organizes memories and information you learned that day. At the same time, your body is repairing and rebuilding itself.

My Tips for Getting Quality Sleep:

- Transition from your day by lying down in your bed at least thirty minutes to an hour before the time you need to be asleep.

- Make the room as dark as possible.

- Don't eat for at least an hour before bedtime.

- Keep a consistent bedtime. Try to go to sleep within one hour of that time each night.

- Use sound to drown out noises that can wake you up.

- Make the room cold.

- Stop using your phone or watching TV one hour before bed.

- Read or listen to audiobooks while in bed to help you relax.

Mental Recovery

I have struggled with depression and anger issues my whole life. When I started working out, I felt better, but it wasn't until I started to slowly incorporate mental recovery strategies like daily meditation, practicing gratitude, and spending time in nature that I started to really notice a difference in how I felt and stopped reacting to situations and started responding to them.

I was never into self-care. I always thought meditation was for monks, but once I opened myself up to the idea that it could be helpful, and when I really tried to let all my thoughts go and focus on my breathing, I did start to feel its power.

Taking the time to help my mental state was hard at first. Growing up, I felt pressure from society to be a "man", that meant to be tough and not talk about my feelings, but as I get older and wiser, I realize that we all need to talk about how we feel in a constructive way and do things for ourselves to improve our mental health and so we can have closure and enjoy life to its fullest.

<u>Gratitude</u>

I recently read a book called *Finding Gratitude in H.O.P.E.* by Rusty Williams. Rusty is a friend of mine who I met in a book writing class—the class that inspired me to write this book in fact. In his book, he talks about how he finds gratitude while living with a debilitating spinal cord tumor. If he can find things to be grateful for, then you can too.

When you take the time to think of all the good things in your life, like your loved ones, your health (if you're reading this, you're still alive), your experiences, or your friends, you put things in perspective and focus on the good things in your life. This will help you feel better when you're feeling down and will make you appreciate your life.

Community

We are social creatures by nature and require positive interactions and relationships with others to be fulfilled. It is important to surround yourself with kind, loving, and supportive people that will lift you up when you are down and be there to celebrate the good times, too.

Your community could consist of family, friends, or coworkers, and the time you spend with them should be in person as much as possible. Texting or talking to someone on your phone is okay, but the magic happens when you're in the same room, so to speak. You need to be able to feel their energy and pick up on their nonverbal cues. These shared experiences will strengthen your bond and bring you closer together.

Some people get community from their religion, others from shared hobbies. You might have a big family, and that might be enough. However you find people to share your life with, make sure they are worthy of you. They should be respectful of you and your boundaries and willing to listen when you need to vent.

If you need more community in your life, try going to some meetups (Meetup.com) in your area, or do more things you like to do and be open to meeting new people. Be yourself, and the right people will gravitate toward you.

<u>Nature</u>

Nature is the best! We came from nature. We are animals, after all. Sometimes, we need to get back into it to ground ourselves, rid ourselves of negative energy, and re-energize our minds and bodies.

Ever since I was a child, when I would get upset, my mom would tell me, "Go outside and get some fresh air." It always seemed to do the trick. To this day, when I am stressed out, I will go outside, wherever I am, and take a few deep breaths of fresh air to help clear and calm my mind.

Have you heard of forest bathing? It's the Japanese practice of spending time in nature, particularly in forests. This can consist of walking or meditating among trees. There is something about being around trees that can help boost your mood and reduce stress. You have to put your devices away and mindfully experience the sights, sounds, and smells to get the full experience.

Cities are unnatural places, mostly devoid of the plants and animals we evolved with. If you live in a big city, try to find a big park with lots of trees, or take a few hours to go find some nature nearby so you can experience the power of getting back to nature. Make sure you do this safely. Don't expose yourself to extreme weather without the proper gear. Make sure you know where you are at all times so you don't get lost. Be prepared with water and emergency supplies, just in case.

<u>Meditation</u>

I was skeptical of meditation at first. I thought, *How is just sitting there with my eyes shut supposed to help me?* I was dealing with a lot of stress from work, and I didn't know what else to do, so I decided to try a guided meditation.

At first, all these random thoughts kept creeping into my head, but after about five minutes or so, I was able to start focusing on my breathing, and when the ten minutes were up, I felt better. I felt a sense of accomplishment and relief from my stress. I even tried it outside in the sun, and that seemed to boost the effects. I loved the feeling of the wind on my skin and hearing the birds sing. I started meditating every day, and after a few weeks, I noticed that I felt more in control and wasn't just reacting to situations. I also noticed that I had more mental bandwidth to solve problems and deal with difficult situations.

Stress is a huge factor in overall health, and meditation can help reduce stress. It's free, and you can do it anywhere. If you have never meditated before or have fallen out of practice, I would highly recommend you give it a try, even if it's just for five minutes. If you truly make an effort, it will help calm your mind and give you more patience. You can also change your mood or relax simply by doing some deep breathing. Next time you need this, simply take three deep breaths with your eyes closed and see how you feel. You'll feel better, I'm sure of it.

Physical Recovery

Now that you have some ways to help optimize your mental state, let's discuss how to expedite healing your body from stress. Did you know stress can be good for you? When something is hard or "stressful" it is challenging, and this is how we grow.

When you start to use your body in novel ways, you may notice parts of it that do not feel quite right. This is due to the stress you are putting on your body, and it may result in sore or tight muscles, stiff joints, or pain. If an exercise hurts, stop doing it. Then modify it so it doesn't hurt. This kind of pain is different from the discomfort you feel when you're stretching. I'm referring to the bad kind of pain—the kind that does damage to your body, like torn ligaments or tendons.

I struggle constantly with physical recovery—it's in my DNA. I do not know the scientific terminology, but I have weak joints that are susceptible to injury. I have dealt with wrist, shoulder, elbow, and knee issues. I also have a mild case of compartment syndrome. This is when the fascia surrounding the muscles is too tight and constricts the growth of the muscles. I notice it a lot in my calves. I naturally have gigantic calves. If I walk, run, or jump too much, they get really tight and uncomfortable. I have also felt this in my forearms at times. But I was able to overcome all these issues with the tools discussed in this section of the book.

To find long-term success, you'll want to address any issues you experience so you can recover and continue to grow stronger and more resilient. The best advice is to simply not overdo it and allow for rest days in between resistance training so your body has time to repair, rebuild, and heal itself.

Here are the techniques I use to help my body recover:

<u>Hydration</u>

Staying hydrated is one of the easiest and most important things you can do to keep your body functioning properly, like a well-oiled machine. Remember, you are mostly made of water, but that's only half of the equation. Water can only help so much. The game changer is replacing the electrolytes you lose through sweating by adding them to your water. Electrolytes are minerals that carry an electric charge and allow your body to communicate with itself. They help with brain function, muscle contraction, and fluid balance.

Keep in mind that if you eat a mostly whole-food diet, you will definitely need more electrolytes than someone who eats mostly processed foods. You can get them by adding salt to your food or by mixing electrolytes in your water. If you're dehydrated, you won't be able to think clearly or perform at your best, so make sure to drink lots of water and consume electrolytes to stay at peak performance.

<u>Sauna</u>

I like to go in the sauna for twenty-minute sessions after a workout, especially if I have any kind of injury. The heat increases blood circulation and, in turn, speeds up healing. Heat shock proteins are also produced by your body due to the heat stress. These heat shock proteins can reduce oxidative stress, improve cellular function, and make you more comfortable in hot environments. They can also play a role in longevity.

Besides all of the physical health benefits of saunas, I really enjoy the challenge of staying in there for an extended period of time. Your body is saying, "Get the heck out of here; you're going to die," but I know I'm okay, and overcoming that feeling is rewarding. And I love how relaxed I feel when I get out. This is one of those challenging things I mentioned—it goes a long way in building confidence and overall happiness.

If you don't have access to a sauna, find a hot place to go and sweat it out for a bit. This could be in a car on a hot day or in a small room with a space heater. You could also wear a sweater on a warm day. Whether you're in a sauna or a hot car, do it responsibly. Don't overdo it, and make sure to hydrate after or during.

Isolated Heat

Heat pads or packs are another tool I use for sore or stiff muscles. It's an old-school method, but it works well and is more practical than a sauna. It does not have all the benefits of a sauna, but it can help with healing and pain relief. The heat draws in the blood and promotes circulation, which expedites healing and relaxes tight tissues.

You can use an electric heat pad or an ice pack filled with hot water. You can even make your own by putting rice in a cloth bag and microwaving it.

Cold Exposure therapy

Exposing your body to cold temperatures helps to reduce inflammation by promoting blood circulation and forcing your body to create cold shock proteins, which have similar effects as heat shock proteins, with the exception that they help you adapt to cold environments rather than hot ones. Cold exposure can also make you feel alive, by releasing endorphins, prolong your life, and present a challenge for you to overcome.

The best way to do cold exposure therapy is to use a cold plunge pool, but if you don't have access to one, you could go into a cold body of water, take a cold shower, or go outside when it's cold with minimal clothing.

Start slow by doing it for a minute, and then work up to three minutes. That is all you need to gain all of the positive effects and experience a feeling of bliss that can last for hours. As always, use caution and don't expose yourself to extreme cold temperatures for extended periods of time.

My favorite time to go into a cold plunge pool is immediately after I get out of a session in the sauna.

<u>Cupping</u>

Cupping is an ancient practice from Chinese medicine that's still used today. It's a great tool for sore or tight muscles, and it's another way to promote blood circulation. Have you noticed a trend? Improved blood circulation helps with so many ailments in our bodies and is key for physical recovery. Originally, a bamboo cup was heated with a flame and placed on the skin. The temperature difference creates a vacuum, and the suction is what helps to stretch and loosen the affected tissues and draw in the blood. It's also said to draw toxins out of the blood. There are a few different types of cups and techniques, and they don't involve a flame.

I use silicone cups for several reasons. One, they work great; two, they don't require a pump; and three, they're portable, so I can take them with me when I travel. I put them on sore or tight muscles by pushing down on the top, placing them on my skin, and when I let go, a vacuum is created. I leave them on for about ten minutes, and when I take them off, I feel relief from the affected area, plus I get the added bonus of having cool circular marks left on my skin to show how badass I am. They can be painful to use, but they're so worth it when you have tight, cramped muscles.

Active cupping is always painful, but it can really get in there and free up tense muscles. You do this by adding massage oil to your skin and moving the suctioned cup around. It's like a deep tissue massage and really helps me with my tight calves.

Massage

Massage can be a mental and physical recovery tool. Whether it's from a hydro-massage bed, a massage gun, or a masseuse, it can be very relaxing and help work out the lactic acid that builds up in your muscles after strenuous exercise. It can also be relaxing and make you feel good, so if you're stressed out or have tightness that you need worked out, take the extra time and get a massage however you can.

Stretching

The older you get, the more important stretching becomes. I would recommend stretching at any age, not only to improve flexibility but also to warm up your body to avoid injury. It only takes one move to injure yourself, so why not get some insurance on your health by doing some stretching before and after any exercise? You can find a video online to guide you through a quick stretching routine or do it intuitively.

Foam rolling can be a great way to get a deep stretch. The more it hurts, the more you need it. Sometimes, when my calves get really tight, foam rolling is the only way to get relief. If you're tight in a specific area, don't just focus on that alone; pay attention to the parts of your body that connect to that area as well. For example, when my calves hurt, I make sure to pay attention to my hamstrings, hip flexors, and ankles to loosen up the whole lower leg.

There are lots of videos online that can help you with specific areas that you want to focus on, but make sure to do a full-body stretch as often as you can. When your body is loose, you are less likely to injure yourself.

Practicing mental and physical recovery will take you to the next level of overall health. Your body/mind connection is a real thing, and one affects the other. If you're stressed out, anxious, or depressed, it will have physical negative effects on your body. And if you're not properly nourishing or exercising your body, it will negatively affect your mind.

I didn't start my health journey using these recovery practices. I learned them along the way, and when I started to incorporate them into my routine, I discovered that they play a critical role in helping me strengthen my mind and my body.

Now it's your turn to try some of these practices. Pick one idea from each of these areas, go do it, and see how you feel. If it's not for you, keep trying different things until you find something that works for you and makes you feel good. The whole point of all of this is to feel good and enjoy your time on Earth to the fullest.

CHAPTER 12:
STARTING YOUR HEALTH JOURNEY

In Chapter 1, I told you that if you started to eat the proper amount of protein, you would start to make healthier food choices, feel better, and have more energy. It's true; if all you did was eat more whole protein and didn't follow anything else I have written about, you would experience all those things. But if you slowly start to incorporate proper nutrition, exercise, and recovery into your life, you will experience all these benefits and a lot more.

I was able to successfully turn these strategies into habits, and I am the healthiest I have ever been in my life, and I'm just shy of forty. I feel great, especially on the days I take the time to meditate, work out, and eat well! I have so much energy I don't even need to drink coffee to get through the day—I still do because I like it, but I don't rely on it like I used to. You need to be able to do the things you like and not deprive yourself. If these things are not healthy, do them in moderation or find ways to make them better for you.

If you don't know where to start, I would recommend you start with a mindfulness practice if you're not already implementing one. For example, start meditating in the morning and setting intentions for your day. You will be surprised how simply taking some time for yourself to be present and expressing what you want will improve your mood and give you more confidence to change the things you want to change.

Another place to start is getting enough sleep. I know it's easier said than done, but if you prioritize getting the right amount of high-quality sleep, it will allow your brain to process new ideas and work better, allowing you to make better choices and be stronger in your decision-making. Do whatever it takes to get enough rest. If you're not well-rested, you will struggle with your health regardless of how well you eat or how much you work out.

All said, to get the fastest and most dramatic results, you'll need to find out what foods are right for your body and avoid eating the ones that aren't. The easiest way to do this is to go carnivore. It's essentially an elimination diet. Once you have been only eating meat for a month, you can start adding other whole foods to your diet to see how they affect you. If you're a non-meat person, avoid processed foods at all costs. I know it's hard, but that's the price you have to pay when you don't eat the food your body evolved to eat. You will have to make sure you're getting enough whole proteins and eating a variety of plant foods so you get all the nutrients you need.

Start walking more. If you walk ten thousand steps a day, walk twenty thousand. Walking is low-impact and gets you outside, so you can take advantage of all the benefits of sunlight on your skin and fresh air in your lungs.

It's important to have a well-rounded health and fitness regimen, and by slowly incorporating the strategies discussed in this book and developing them into habits, you will find long-term success.

You can do this!

Make sure to take it one step at a time, and always be open to adapting to whatever life throws at you. Adapt and overcome, as the marines say. By choosing one thing to start with and sticking with it, you will make progress. The key is to keep your momentum moving forward.

Don't try to start doing everything you've learned all at once; it's too much. It's easy to get overwhelmed and feel discouraged if you take on too much at once. Whatever you do, don't give up, and if you fall off your horse, dust yourself off, take a deep breath, and get back on.

Once you master one strategy, try implementing another, and if it's not working for you, switch it out for another one. Eventually, you will find what works for you, and you can be proud of yourself for doing your best. You can experience the benefits of *Living the Protein Lifestyle* for yourself if you take that first step and continue working on yourself.

CHAPTER 13:
Si Se Puede

It's been four years now since I started replacing my bad habits with good ones. I still have a few that I'm working on, and that's okay because I'm still trying. This is the most important piece of advice I can give you: No matter how many times you stray from your goals, never give up; keep trying. Make small changes, and over time, you will see big results.

I find myself craving whole foods and enjoy staying active. I was depressed and felt bad about how I treated my body, but now that I'm *Living the Protein Lifestyle*, I'm happier, and I feel good about myself (when I follow my own advice). I still have my bad days, and that's okay.

I lost fifty pounds in two years, and I managed to keep the weight I lost off despite having a knee injury and subsequent surgery that took me several months to recover from. I still could lose another twenty pounds, so I'm going to continue to eat lots of meat and whole foods, workout at least a few times a week, and go for walks with our dogs every day. These habits have drastically improved my quality of life by making my body stronger and more resilient and giving me more energy to enjoy my life. I feel good most days, and my wife quite often comments on how good I look.

I still allow myself to drink Coke (mini cans), eat chocolate ice cream, have an adult beverage, or smoke a little weed from time to time, but I do my best to limit those types of behaviors because I know they are not the best for me. As far as I know, we only get one shot at this thing called life, and I believe you should be able to do what you want as long as it is in moderation, and you aren't harming anyone.

Find a healthy balance in everything you do and occasionally allow yourself to do things that aren't the best for you. You'll have to put in the work the rest of the time so you can feel your best and avoid injuries and diseases, but you should not deprive yourself of the things you like to do.

I'd like to tell you a story about a woman named Sally who struggled with health issues her whole life but after only a week of eating lean beef, chicken breast, some pork, and a few select vegetables, started to feel better and noticed her symptoms starting to lessen in severity.

When Sally was a young girl, she was diagnosed with Raynaud's disease, a circulatory disorder that affects the blood vessels in the extremities. There's no cure for this, so all she could do was manage the symptoms.

In her late thirties, she started feeling lethargic all the time, to the point where she started falling asleep while driving. She was also suffering from irritable bowel syndrome, hair loss, and debilitating migraine headaches. She told me, "Even my bones would hurt, and I had trouble walking."

Sally went to her general practitioner and was diagnosed with lupus, an autoimmune disease that can affect many different parts of the body. Her doctor prescribed her an anti-inflammatory, a corticosteroid, an antimalarial, and last but not least, the dreaded immunosuppressant. If this wasn't enough, the doctor also told her, "Try to avoid triggers like sunlight exposure and manage your symptoms to reduce the risk of flare-ups."

This regimen helped a little, but she couldn't live like this, and she didn't know what else to do. Sally was doing research on how to help herself and came across a lecture on hyperthyroidism. She felt that everything the speaker was saying described what she was dealing with, so she contacted the speaker and scheduled an appointment. This doctor told her she most likely had hypothyroidism and recommended she do a food allergy test. So she did and discovered that she was allergic or sensitive to almost everything she was eating, which included dairy, wheat, and soy. So, she started only eating meat as an elimination diet, and within a week, she started feeling better.

Sally continued her meat-centric diet, avoided the foods that didn't agree with her, started working out regularly, and started meditating daily to deal with her stress. One year later, all her symptoms were gone, and she felt better than ever. She was still eating a meat-heavy diet but was able to slowly add more foods back into her diet.

Sally is proof that making protein the center of your diet and adding a little exercise to your life can go a long way toward improving your health. You can take control of your health, too! Get a food allergy test or try an elimination diet to find out what foods are right for you.

Eating right is not the only factor: mental recovery is critical. If you don't care enough about yourself to take care of your body, then you will not be successful. You need to do this for you and no one else.

By following the simple tips I have shared with you, you can find success. Meditate daily, get some physical exercise most days, and most important of all to living that protein lifestyle is to make protein the main focus of every meal!

Pick one of the concepts in this book that really calls to you and start doing that as soon as possible. Once you begin, it will jump-start your health journey, and you'll start to feel better. Slowly continue to add more concepts to your routine until you are the embodiment of the protein lifestyle, and you will feel your best. It's not easy, but you are worth it, and the longer you stick with it, the easier it will get. If you can form these strategies into habits, then after a while, you won't even have to think about it; they'll become another part of your daily routine.

You may find it hard to get started, but once you do, you'll notice positive changes. Start slow, and don't be too hard on yourself. You will be amazed at how happy you can be by just changing a few things and making informed choices about the food you eat. We all struggle with health, but now you know what you can do to make a difference.

You may not be able to stick with it one hundred percent of the time, and that is totally okay. As long as you keep trying, you will make progress and find success. Take a deep breath and go be your best self! Si se puede (Yes, you can).

Are you ready to start feeling and looking your best?

Do you want a step-by-step guide on how to improve your health?

Get the new *Protein Lifestyle Workbook*!

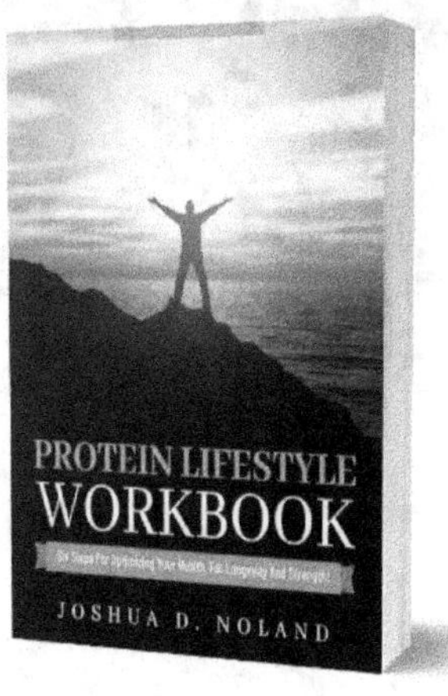

This workbook shows you exactly how to set yourself up for long-term health success with a detailed step-by-step guide that is easy to follow, ensuring you take the actions you need to start making lasting changes to optimize your health at your own pace and with confidence.

ProteinLifestyleWorkbook.com

www.ingramcontent.com/pod-product-compliance
Lightning Source LLC
Chambersburg PA
CBHW050729260726
48661CB00001B/148